THE
HORMONE
REVOLUTION
WEIGHT-LOSS PLAN

Dear HSIN mei,

Best of wishes!

K. Chris, MD

3/03

THE HORMONE REVOLUTION WEIGHT-LOSS PLAN

Harness
the Power
of Your
Fat-Burning
Hormones

KARLIS ULLIS, M.D.
with JOSHUA SHACKMAN, PH.D.

AVERY
a member of
Penguin Putnam Inc.

a member of
Penguin Putnam Inc.
375 Hudson Street
New York, NY 10014
www.penguinputnam.com

Library of Congress Cataloging-in-Publication Data

Ullis, Karlis.
The hormone revolution weight-loss plan : harness the power
of your fat-burning hormones / by Karlis Ullis with Joshua Shackman.
p.   cm.
Includes bibliographical references and index.
ISBN 1-58333-135-2
1. Weight loss—Endocrine aspects.   2. Fat—Metabolism.   I. Shackman, Joshua.   II. Title.
RM222.2.U43   2003
613.7—dc21   2002072815

Printed in the United States of America
1   3   5   7   9   10   8   6   4   2

This book is printed on acid-free paper. ∞

Book design by Stephanie Huntwork

The Hormone Revolution Weight-Loss Plan is dedicated to all of my patients and athletes for their many devoted hours of exercise and correct eating. Without their enthusiasm and spirit, the conception and completion of this book would have not been possible.

—K.U.

ACKNOWLEDGMENTS

I would first like to thank my literary agent, Harvey Klinger, and my editors, Laura Shepherd and Kristen Jennings, all of whom believed in this project from the beginning and provided me with useful advice and support. I would also like to thank my expert team of nutritional specialists: Anna Brantman, M.S.; Rehan Jalali, B.S.; Mason Panetti, C.N.C.; and Cristiana Paul, M.S., who provided me with much technical assistance during the writing of this book. Nazy Emami contributed research assistance for the initial stages of the book. Jason Grace of DirectEdgeMedia.com provided us with the diagrams in the exercise appendix. I would like to thank Dr. Frederick Hatfield, whose "Dr. Squat" webpage and other materials were a tremendous resource for information and the diagrams on weight training. I also benefited greatly from the many lively debates and discussions with the Los Angeles Gerontology Research Group and with the Longevity Rx anti-aging discussion group. I would like to thank all the active members of these organizations, as they provided me with useful commentary and food for thought while I was writing this book.

—K.U.

CONTENTS

PREFACE   xi

INTRODUCTION   1

ONE

Fat-Burning Hormones: The Simple Guide   5

TWO

The Hormone Revolution Exercise Plan   19

THREE

The Hormone Revolution Eating Plan   39

FOUR

The Hormone Revolution Supplement Plan   96

FIVE

Monitoring Your Success   114

SIX

Lifestyle and Aging   129

SEVEN

Lifelong Benefits   145

Creating a Personalized Program   156

APPENDIX I

Basic Exercise Instructions   158

APPENDIX II

Information Resources   167

APPENDIX III

Expertise   174

SELECTED REFERENCES   177

INDEX   185

PREFACE

I have been blessed to have a career in medicine that has allowed me to work with people of all ages and all walks of life. It is through this long experience that I became aware of the extreme importance of hormones to health and fitness. From my work with children, elite athletes, and middle-aged and elderly people, I have found that maintaining a proper balance of hormones is necessary for sustaining good health, high energy levels, and a lean and fit body.

My career has taken many interesting twists and turns since my initial residency training and faculty clinical appointment at the Department of Pediatrics at the UCLA School of Medicine. But I have always thought pediatrics and working with growing children was the right place to start my medical career. Children are usually born healthy and with lots of energy. It is only as they are exposed to unhealthy lifestyles that they begin to suffer from the adult problems of poor nutrition and obesity. I learned that the challenge of good health and medicine is to maintain a youthful and energetic state for an entire lifetime.

While working in pediatrics, I extensively researched the problem of growth hormone deficiency in children, an oftentimes traumatic blow to a child's self-esteem. I learned that growth hormone, among other hormones, not only has tremendous effects in stimulating growth in children but also increases energy levels and reduces body fat for people of all ages. The knowledge of the effects of growth hormone that I gained from working with children would later become extremely valuable as I took on new challenges in medicine.

My next area of interest and study was sports medicine. Achieving optimum human performance is quite a challenge, since it requires a determination to stay strong and fit in the face of many obstacles. I couldn't help noticing that many of the hardest-working athletes were often the ones who sabotaged their health and performance the most. Unknowingly, they fell victim to improper exercise and eating habits (including timing) that led to hormonal imbalances and loss of strength.

The athletes I worked with were not stupid. Many of them had almost encyclopedic knowledge of exercise and nutrition. What they lacked was an understanding of the big picture—an overall knowledge of human physiology as a complete system. Some of the most experienced athletes often overexercised and overtrained, thereby destroying their strength and disrupting their hormones in the process.

In order to stay fit, athletes need to maintain healthy habits that will sustain a stable hormone system. From working with athletes, I learned that proper hormone balancing requires an overall lifestyle approach that includes short but effective exercise sessions, proper rest and relaxation time, and a well-conceived diet plan. Rather than wasting all their energy on putting 120 percent into their training, athletes who follow this balanced program perform the best in the long run. This balanced approach has been a big success with the athletes I have worked with on six different Olympic teams as well as with elite athletes at UCLA and many in professional ranks.

After working first with children, then with athletes in their twenties and early thirties, the next logical step in my journey through medicine and time was to work with middle-aged and elderly people. Until recently, this field of medicine only concerned itself with geriatrics, which focuses primarily on learning how to cope and manage the problems of aging. I decided instead to become a pioneer in the field of gerontology—the study of the prevention of the adverse symptoms of aging and the promotion of a healthy, robust longevity.

I have never agreed with my medical peers who think the medical problems associated with aging are inevitable, natural facts of life. Instead, I have always viewed them as the cumulative effects of an unhealthy lifestyle that can be beat if the right steps are taken. I have found that hormone balancing throughout a lifetime is one of the most important factors in fighting the effects of aging.

My years of diverse medical practice and study precipitated my foundation of the innovative Sports Medicine and Anti-Aging Medical Group in Santa Monica, California. I have taken a unique approach in my clinic by combining the latest medical research with my own years of experience in sports medicine and aging to help people fight fatigue, increase their sexual interest and function, and improve the shape of their bodies. Through my work there, I have found that the same concepts of staying strong and balancing your hormones are just as effective for older people as they are for young athletes. Keeping a strong body and maintaining a youthful balance of hormones is the best prescription for optimum health, regardless of your age.

Through my years of work and research, I have become increasingly concerned about obesity—an epidemic disease that is running rampant across our country and around the world. While many people understand the impact that calories, food, and exercise have on their health, they rarely apply this knowledge appropriately to stay lean and healthy. Far too many people are ignorant of the broad impact that hormones have on their bodies, from determining body shape to affecting fat storage and muscle growth. The only way to achieve lasting fitness and weight loss is to implement habits that allow your body to maintain a healthy balance of hormones.

My agent, publisher, and coauthor all urged me to make this a diet book.

But, to me, this book is much more than that. I consider it to be a manual that will lead you through the newest branch of medicine that I call "lifestyle medicine." I am excited to present in a single volume a simple plan for life that an average person with limited medical knowledge can easily understand and follow.

The fact that the Hormone Revolution Weight-Loss Plan will result in weight loss is really just a side effect of healthy living. My real intent in writing this book is to help you achieve overall optimum health while extending your life span while enhancing your quality of life. With the proper synchronization, the three primary elements of the Hormone Revolution program—exercise, diet, and supplements—will work integrally with one another in order to achieve your healthful new lifestyle. Once these steps are in place, you will begin to feel the lasting benefits beyond basic weight loss, including improved muscle strength, increased libido, longevity, relief from many problems of aging, and more. This book will take you through every step of the Hormone Revolution Weight-Loss Plan, arming you with the weapons you need to lose fat and avoid destructive patterns and leading you to a more hormonally healthful life.

INTRODUCTION

It was my pleasure to review this much-needed, indispensable guide to fitness for people of all ages, *The Hormone Revolution Weight-Loss Plan: Harness the Power of Your Fat-Burning Hormones.* As a fitness professional, I am always interested in the latest research on how to get energized, stay lean, and build muscle while maintaining a disease-free and robust life. But also as a baby boomer, I am particularly concerned with the more practical aspects of maintaining fitness, health, and strength as I enter midlife. Dr. Ullis combines the sports science knowledge similar to what I have used in my competitive training with a practical weight-loss and fitness program that he has developed through his years of clinical experience. Together, these elements provide easy-to-understand information on how people at any fitness level can attain a slim, fit body for a lifetime.

Dr. Ullis and I both have worked in the professional fitness arena—he as a sports medicine doctor to athletes, and I as a champion bodybuilder. But I am most pleased that now we are working toward a more universal health goal of applying our specialized experience to help the millions of people trying so hard to lose fat and weight. As I lecture on fitness and host fitness television shows, I look forward to sharing the invaluable information that Dr. Ullis provides in this book—information that so many people struggling with weight loss desperately need to know.

I agree wholeheartedly with Dr. Ullis that weight training is extremely important for the success of any long-term weight-loss plan. Many women are afraid that lifting weights will make them overly muscular and masculine-looking. Even some men say that they don't want to lift weights too much because they don't want to get "too big" or bulky. But I have been telling women and men alike for many years that they do not need to be afraid of weight training. Only a tiny percentage of people has the genetics to become "overly muscular," very few of them women. Contrary to what you may believe, if you do not weight train properly while trying to lose weight, you will sabotage your program completely. You will lose muscle rather than fat, and this will make you weaker and dramatically slow down your metabolism. The drug-free weight-training and eating program in this book will help you achieve a lean, healthy, and strong look that is attractive for both men and women!

The most unique aspect of this book is the information about how you can correctly exercise and eat in order to boost your fat-burning hormones without the use of drugs. Just to understand the alternatives to hormone replacement therapy presented in this book gives hope to those of us who may not want to take medication, opting instead to go through life on a drug-free path. I have seen far too many women fail their diets and weight-loss programs with synthetic hormone replacement drugs that only lead to bloating and unnecessary weight gain. We all need to know the alternatives to prescription medication, and *The Hormone Revolution Weight-Loss Plan* is a valuable one. We do have choices.

I am pleased that Dr. Ullis refers to his book not as a "diet" book but rather as a complete lifestyle plan. In my book *Cory Everson's LifeBalance* (Perigee, 1998), I discuss the importance of balancing proper eating habits, proper exercise, and stress reduction. Too many diet books will lead readers to engage in extreme and destructive behaviors, such as starvation dieting, hours of aerobics, and sleeplessness. I have been known to joke that "*diet* is a four-letter word." Most diet plans are doomed to failure. But *The Hormone Revolution Weight-Loss Plan* emphasizes healthy eating habits rather than starvation dieting, moderate exercise rather than exhaustive overtraining, and healthy sleep and stress reduction instead of imposing undue strain on your life and body. These recommendations are a surefire recipe for success.

I applaud Dr. Ullis for bringing some much-needed, scientifically based concepts for weight loss to the public. We can only win the war on obesity by making the public more educated on how to lead a healthy, balanced life. *The Hormone Revolution Weight-Loss Plan* is an invaluable addition to the world of long-term fitness and weight loss.

—CORY EVERSON

Six-time Ms. Olympia and renowned health and fitness expert

ONE

FAT-BURNING HORMONES: THE SIMPLE GUIDE

FAT LOSS, NOT WEIGHT LOSS

Your body is designed to resist fat loss. In the early days of mankind, the ability to store fat was essential to survival. Primitive man never knew when his next meal would be and needed a healthy storage of fat in order to survive for long periods of time without food. To your body, fat is essential to survival, whereas muscle is a luxury that it can burn away.

Thousands of years of evolution have turned our bodies into efficient fat-storage machines that resist weight loss—we hold on to fat and must work hard to build muscle. But, in modern society, food is not scarce, and we are tempted by cheap and plentiful junk food everywhere we go. To combat your body's tendency to store fat, you must incorporate a precise weight-loss program that will target your fat stores while preserving muscle.

Eat less and exercise, and, yes, you will lose weight. But another factor is at work: When you exercise, your hormones determine what kind of weight you are losing, muscle or fat. Muscle preservation is a major concern for dieters. Muscle burns calories not only when you are exercising but also when you are at rest. Therefore, the more muscle you have, the more potential for fat burning. Unfortunately for dieters, due to our evolutionary history, simply eating less will actually cause your hormones to signal your body to burn your muscle while leaving your fat stores intact. With less muscle, your metabolism will slow down, and fat loss will become all the more difficult. The reality of dieting is that limiting your intake of certain foods can actually make you fatter!

The good news is that, with the right combination of exercises and foods, you can ensure that almost all of your weight loss comes from fat rather than muscle. Some foods, such as proteins, for example, which are highly unlikely to be stored as fat, will help build and maintain muscle mass. And careful planning of the time that you consume some foods, such as carbohydrates—which can be stored as fat or muscle, depending on when you eat them—can aid in both fat burning and muscle preservation. You will learn in the next two chapters that a carefully planned exercise program in conjunction with your diet will influence hormones such as testosterone to help you burn fat without muscle loss. In fact, many people on my program actually gain muscle. The key, as always, is strict hormone regulation.

HARNESSING YOUR HORMONES

Hormones are extremely powerful substances. You have probably heard your doctor talk about hormones, but do you really know what they do or how important they are? Hormones are chemical messengers in your body through which organs communicate with one another. Nearly every bodily function requires a signal from a hormone produced in your body. There are hormones that determine our gender; there are hormones that make you tired and others that give you energy; and there are hormones that cause you to store fat and others that dissolve it.

While a complete description of the hundreds of hormones in your body is beyond the scope of this book, there are two key systems of hormones that are worth discussing in terms of weight loss—the sex hormone system and the insulin system. These two systems, along with the human growth hormone, are the most influential hormones in weight loss. Different foods and exercises cause chain reactions within these systems that affect functions throughout your body, from energy and appetite to broader lifestyle elements such as libido, sleep, and aging. The wrong reactions within these hormone systems can negatively impact the operation of all of these functions and can actually promote weight gain and overall ill health. Throughout this book, you will learn how to stimulate these hormone systems with exercise, diet, supplements, and lifestyle choices in order to influence reactions that will allow you to maximize the health and weight-loss benefits of a balanced hormone system.

The Sex Hormone System

I am sure you are familiar with the basic sex hormones testosterone and estrogen. Because testosterone is known primarily as the male sex hormone, and estrogen as the female hormone, many are surprised to find that each is found in both sexes. While most people are familiar with the masculinizing or feminizing effects of these hormones, very few are aware of the extremely powerful effects they can have—whether you are male or female—on fat burning and fat storage.

Estrogen, for example, has potent effects on fat storage. The fact that women have a level of estrogen higher than that in men is one key reason women naturally have more body fat. Estrogen not only promotes fat storage, it can also make losing weight and fat much more difficult. In fact, farmers often fatten up their livestock by injecting them with estrogen. Synthetic estrogens commonly used in hormone replacement therapies and birth control pills are often fat promoting as well. Women prescribed any form of estrogen, especially synthetic forms, should be aware that these drugs can actually be counterproductive to women's health by promoting weight gain.

Testosterone, on the other hand, has powerful effects that stimulate fat burning, giving younger men a natural advantage over women when it comes to losing fat. You've probably noticed that men under thirty can shed pounds quickly and without much effort. Teenage boys, in particular, who have very high levels of testosterone, can eat large amounts of food with minimal fat gain. Testosterone promotes muscle growth and preservation, which results in increases in the amount of calories burned even while resting. The same hormone that gives young men their strong sex drive also helps them stay lean.

As we get older and mature past our reproductive age, our sex hormone levels naturally drop. From a biological perspective, this is due to that fact that for thousands of years humans lived only to the age of thirty or forty, reproducing in their early teens. Today, while our life spans have greatly increased to double that of our ancestors, our prime reproductive age still passes relatively early in our lives—when we are in our twenties. From that age onward, our sex hormone levels gradually decline. This is unfortunate, as sex hormones not only assist in reproduction but also in promoting energy, strong bones, fat burning, and muscle building—things also often associated with youth.

For aging men, rising levels of estrogen in their bodies compound the disadvantage of the loss of testosterone. Some men in their fifties actually have more estrogen in their systems than women of the same age! This combination can lead to increased fat and weight gain and can also make it very difficult to lose excess fat. As men age and body fat begins to accumulate, levels of aromatase, an enzyme that converts testosterone to estrogen, increase. These higher estrogen levels and lowered testosterone levels boost production of aromatase even further, making weight loss increasingly difficult.

While young women do produce small amounts of testosterone in their bodies (although minuscule compared to levels in young men), which help them to maintain lean bodies, postmenopausal women generally have extremely low testosterone levels. This decrease in testosterone partially explains why women often experience dramatic weight gain after menopause. The loss of fat-burning, muscle-building testosterone can make weight loss close to impossible for many aging women.

Winners and Losers

Studies have shown some very interesting phenomena in terms of sex hormone reactions to the environment. During a soccer game, fans of both teams will experience an increase in testosterone levels. At the end of the game, fans of the winning team will experience an even greater increase in testosterone levels, while the testosterone levels in fans of the losing team will drop back down to normal. Similarly, men competing for the attention of a woman also experience an increase in testosterone, with the man winning the woman's favor maintaining higher levels and the loser's levels returning to normal. Testosterone levels in women increase during ovulation, motivating them to have sex and reproduce right before their fertility reaches its peak. The biological reason for this is that your sex hormones are priming you for reproduction during times of elation, but you can learn how to provoke these increases through exercise and diet to take advantage of testosterone's fat-burning power.

What these studies illustrate is that a key to boosting your testosterone levels is to be a "winner," not necessarily in terms of sports or reproduction but in terms of lifestyle choices. On the Hormone Revolution program, you can influence your hormone levels by participating in "winning" activities such as short but intense weight-lifting sessions and by eating several small, balanced meals throughout the day. Because these activities raise your testosterone levels (as you will learn more about in the next two chapters), you will be able to take advantage of testosterone's benefits—muscle stimulation, increased energy levels, and an enhanced libido.

I have found that most other diet and exercise programs work against you by promoting "losing" activities. The combination of too much aerobics and starvation diets that deprive your body of fat or carbohydrates wears your body down, causing testosterone levels to drop and valuable muscle to be burned. In the long run, you will likely get fatter as a result of following a poor diet and exercise program. But my Hormone Revolution program is designed to give you a winning lifestyle that allows you to harness the power of your sex hormones to promote fitness.

The Insulin System

The sex hormone system is not the only hormone system that has powerful effects on fat burning. Those of you familiar with low-carbohydrate diets are probably aware of the importance of the hormone insulin on weight loss. Many of the low-carbohydrate diets such as the Zone or the Atkins diet focus almost solely on the role of insulin in fat loss and fat storage. While I agree that proper insulin management is very important for losing fat, I find most low-carbohydrate diets greatly oversimplify the issue.

Insulin levels rise in your body after you eat as it removes the excess sugar from your blood and stores it in your muscles and other cells to be used as energy. Carbohydrates in particular provoke strong insulin responses because they are quickly absorbed into your blood as sugar, rapidly raising your glucose levels. Once your body has stored enough glucose in your muscles and other cells for fuel, insulin works to divert the excess into fat stores. Advocates of low-carb diets are correct in pointing out that eating carbohydrates can result in an increase in insulin that can make you fatter. And because one of insulin's other main roles is to protect and preserve your fat stores, increased levels also can make fat burning nearly impossible. I agree that insulin's response to carbohydrates and many other foods can promote fat storage, but only if you eat incorrectly.

The typical American diet is overstimulating our insulin hormonal system. Many of the foods we eat (not just carbohydrates) are almost toxic to our bodies and are driving us toward obesity and, increasingly, diabetes. Processed foods, fast foods, and junk foods are loaded with unhealthy fats and processed starches. Starches often overstimulate our insulin systems, which lead can to diabetes over time. Unhealthy fats, such as the synthetic trans-fatty acids found in most junk foods, also lead to poor insulin function. Insulin poisoning from eating too many unhealthy foods has contributed to the 33 percent increase in the obesity rate over the last ten years. The diabetes rate also is steadily increasing. One study forecasts that the overall diabetes rate in the United States will increase by 165 percent over the next fifty years!

If harnessed properly, however, insulin will not store the carbohydrates you eat as fat. The insulin system reacts in different ways at different times of the day to different types of foods. In fact, if eaten at the proper times, the carbohydrates you eat can be stored as sugar in your muscles to help fuel your exercise program. If you attune your diet to regulate your insulin levels, you can minimize the fat-storage effects of insulin while promoting the appetite-suppressing powers of the entire insulin system.

I often call the insulin system "the appetite-regulating hormone system" because of its powerful effects on your appetite. Excessively high insulin levels result in dangerously low blood sugar. Your body will perceive that it is actually starving, causing it to compensate by triggering an increase in your appetite. Improper eating and exercise timing can cause your appetite to become uncontrollable. The urge to binge eat is frequently caused by poor management of your insulin system, a problem that this program can obliterate.

Growth Hormone

Human growth hormone is an important trigger for normal growth in children, hence its name. But growth hormone also can have some positive effects in adults. Studies and my own clinical experience have shown that growth hormone can be highly effective for burning fat if used correctly. Growth hormone is a "fat mobilizer" that signals enzymes in your body to preferentially burn fat instead of carbohydrates or muscle—it actually alters the action of fat-storing enzymes so that they will burn fat instead. It also plays a fundamental role in promoting the growth and repair of vital tissues and organs and, over time, can help build bone mass. As we age, the decline in growth hormone can actually cause us to get fatter, lose bone mass, and make it difficult for our bodies to recover from injuries.

Like other fat-burning hormones, levels of growth hormone tend to drop as you get older. Some people opt to go on growth hormone replacement therapy under the supervision of a medical doctor. While this therapy can be effective for some people, it is also extremely expensive to buy a prescription and requires daily injections. However, on the Hormone Revolution program, this kind of undesirable artificial stimulation is unnecessary. Instead, through proper diet and exercise, you can increase your body's natural production and release of growth hormone to assist in fat burning and building or preserving muscle while avoiding activities that inhibit its production.

METABOLISM

Your metabolism consists of physical and chemical processes in your body through which you dictate how to use energy from the calories in your diet for several functions, including digestion, absorption, elimination, respiration, circulation, and temperature regulation. Your hormones are an integral part of your metabolic system in that they help determine where the calories come from within your body to burn for energy—muscle or fat. If you lower your caloric intake too much (as many diets do), your body's natural survival mechanism will respond by lowering your metabolism in order to preserve the calories you do have. This won't allow you to lose weight or burn fat efficiently, as your body will fight to actually protect the fat and calories.

Thyroid hormone is important in regulating your metabolism: If you don't consume enough calories, your thyroid hormone levels will drop significantly. One way to prevent thyroid levels from dropping while dieting is through the Magic Window Meal (discussed in Chapter 3), which supplies your liver with adequate stores of carbohydrates to help prevent your body from slumping into starvation mode. Maintaining balanced hormones controls your metabolism, ensuring that the calories stored in your body are being utilized to burn fat and control your appetite.

APPETITE

Hunger is probably a dieter's single biggest complaint. Follow most diet plans, and, after a few days, your appetite will become uncontrollable. One reason most diets fail is that they do not take into consideration how different foods stimulate your appetite-regulating hormones. Some foods will cause a hormonal reaction that will send a signal to your brain that your body needs more food. These signals can be so strong that they become almost impossible to resist. No matter how strong-willed you are, eventually you are going to go off your diet and end up binge eating. Once this happens, it is likely that you will end up gaining more weight than you previously lost.

An example of an appetite-regulating hormone is cholecystokinin (CCK), which is released when you eat certain foods—such as various proteins and vegetables—and signals your brain that you have eaten enough. An added benefit of these foods is that they do not stimulate insulin levels or promote fat storage. However, eating foods that boost insulin, such as starchy carbohydrates, may initially make you feel full due to their bulk, but they do not promote the release of CCK and will cause you to become hungry again quickly. This affects your appetite negatively in two ways: (1) It makes you consume more food and calories to feel full, and (2) the insulin stimulation causes your body to store the calories as fat.

Pharmaceutical companies are spending millions of dollars on research to find a drug that mimics the effects of appetite-regulating hormones and effectively suppresses your appetite. The infamous "phen-fen" drug combination was one of the few treatments that was a successful appetite suppressant. Unfortunately, it was also extremely dangerous to your health and ended up being removed from the market.

But you do not need expensive, potentially harmful drugs to control your appetite. Many foods have "druglike" effects on your appetite-regulating hormones. Just as some foods will make you hungrier, others, such as high-fiber vegetables or lean sources of protein, can almost completely suppress your appetite with very few calories. I have carefully developed the diet program in Chapter 3 so that you never have to feel hungry. In fact, I have found that some of the tastiest foods nature has to offer are among the most effective in suppressing your appetite. These are foods that trigger hormonal reactions that signal your brain to stop eating.

HORMONES AND YOUR LIFESTYLE

Our busy and stressful lifestyles also can undermine our fat-burning hormones. You may be aware of the many health hazards of too much stress and not enough sleep. But you may not know that stress and lack of sleep can contribute to obesity and make weight and fat loss more difficult. This topic will be discussed extensively in Chapter 6, but I will give you a brief overview here of the different aspects of your lifestyle that affect your hormones and through them your overall health and fitness.

Stress

When you are under too much stress, your body releases "stress hormones," such as cortisol, which lead to increased muscle loss and fat storage. There are two main types of stress: psychological stress, which results from worrying too much and not taking enough breaks from your hectic lifestyle, and physical stress, which results from smoking, lack of sleep, drinking too much alcohol, and other unhealthy lifestyle choices. Both types of stress will sabotage your fat-burning hormones if you are not careful. Failure to take time to relax is a major reason why dieting can be so difficult.

Medication

Many of the medications prescribed to both men and women for common ailments can disrupt our hormonal systems. These are side effects that are usually ignored or even forgotten by many medical doctors. In many cases, alternative drugs that do not disrupt our hormones are available and will be discussed in Chapter 5.

Sleep

Sleep is extremely important for harnessing your fat-burning hormones. When you sleep, a series of complex chemical messengers in your body signals your brain that more testosterone and human growth hormone production are necessary. Neglecting sleep will disrupt these messengers, denying your body the fat-burning benefits of the increased levels of these important hormones.

Energy

A lack of energy can be a major obstacle to sticking with any weight-loss program that requires exercise such as the Hormone Revolution program. And fatigue doesn't always result from a simple lack of sleep. Many people find that they become more fatigued when they stop exercising for a prolonged period of time, whereas others get worn out from working out too much. As you will learn in the next two chapters, you can combat fatigue through adequate exercise and diet planning that will promote hormone stimulation and boost your energy.

Libido

There is a very strong connection between fat-burning hormones and your libido. Of course, sex hormones have especially potent effects on your libido: If you have a healthy testosterone/estrogen balance, you also will have a healthy libido. As explained later, your libido can be one of the best markers of success while following the Hormone Revolution program. If your libido is low, you are likely sabotaging your fat-burning hormones and are clearly on the wrong path. Conversely, if you are following my program correctly, you can actually increase your libido.

THE HORMONE REVOLUTION
WEIGHT-LOSS PLAN

The delicate balance of the effects of diet, exercise, and supplements on your body's hormones is at the heart of my Hormone Revolution program. You will benefit from my years of working with elite athletes in designing an exercise program for maximum effect and minimal time commitment. In Chapter 2, I will tell you not only *what* exercises to do but also *when* to do them—both extremely important factors in fat burning and fitness.

Once you start exercising, you will find that your dietary habits will improve without much effort. The dietary aspect of this program allows you to lose weight without starvation or cravings. Just as with exercise, the timing of meals and snacks is an extremely important factor that has a tremendous impact on your body's hormones. In Chapter 3, I will take you step by step through my diet program, which is designed to harness the fat-burning power of your hormones. This will include instruction on what to buy at the grocery store, what meals to cook, what to order at restaurants, and even how to schedule your meals throughout the day.

I also will discuss how you may eat starchy carbohydrates forbidden by most low-carbohydrate diet books by carefully coordinating the timing of your exercise with the timing of your meals and thereby create the "Magic Window" period.

After you have your exercise and diet in place, the next important step in the Hormone Revolution program is dietary supplements. In Chapter 4, I will clear up much of the confusion about the numerous supplements widely available at health food stores and supermarkets. This will include a discussion of the vitamins, minerals, and antioxidants that are indispensable to your life functions, help protect you against an often toxic modern life-style, and give your weight-loss program an extra charge.

As mentioned in the preface, this is a complete lifelong lifestyle program. In Chapter 5, I will discuss in more detail how your lifestyle and life cycle affect your fat-burning hormones. Getting proper sleep, minimizing stress, and avoiding hormone-busting medications, chemicals, and other environmental factors are extremely important to the program. Your life cycle (especially menopause and andropause) also has a tremendous impact on your fat-burning hormones. Pay no attention to the doctors who tell you that weight gain, loss of energy, and a declining libido are just natural and inevitable facts of aging. The Hormone Revolution program gives you the tools you need to improve your health for a lifetime.

In Chapter 6, I will explain how the program does more than help you achieve weight loss; it can actually promote longevity and improve your quality of life. Achieving and maintaining hormone balance will help you fight and prevent many diseases, restore youthful energy levels, and improve sexual performance.

Finally, in Chapter 7, I will tell you how to plan and monitor your weight-loss program so you can stay on track and keep making progress until your goals are met. It is now easier than ever to monitor your progress, as we have access to many new and useful technologies. I doubt that modern science will ever come up with a magical invention for weight loss, but it can sure make it much easier to follow my Hormone Revolution program.

Reading this book will only take a few hours of your time, but the information in this book can change your life. So let's get started and join the Hormone Revolution!

TWO

THE HORMONE REVOLUTION
EXERCISE PLAN

BEGINNING YOUR EXERCISE PROGRAM

Before you make any other changes to your daily routine, you should begin your weight-loss program by exercising; it is the essential first step. Exercise is the key to putting your hormones into a fat-burning mode. After that, diet and other lifestyle choices will fall into place quickly.

Controlling the quality of exercise through timing, type, and intensity is central to the Hormone Revolution exercise program. Timing exercise with a proper diet helps release fat-burning, muscle-building hormones to stimulate your workout. The two types of exercise crucial to the program are aerobics and weight lifting, neither of which should be neglected or favored. The level of intensity during your aerobic and weight-lifting sessions in this program is designed to be manageable for even the most stubborn couch potato and guards against overexertion and hormonal burnout.

This program does require you to plan and monitor your exercise more carefully than most others, but the benefits are overwhelming. In this chapter, you will learn how to implement your exercise program, and in Chapter 5 you will learn how to successfully monitor your progress.

Getting Started

The most important step in planning your workout schedule is a very simple one—get started! Unfortunately, this can also be the most difficult part of an exercise program. Below are three methods for overcoming the obstacles to this first crucial step. Once you get started, you will actually have trouble stopping, because you will feel so much better and will have made such tremendous progress.

Method 1: Visit a Doctor or Personal Trainer

Getting the instruction of a well-qualified health professional or a personal trainer is particularly important with this exercise program. It is important to make sure you use the correct technique when weight training so that you get the maximum benefit from the exercise and don't injure yourself or cause back problems. I suggest you visit a doctor or personal trainer and have him or her go over some simple weight-training exercises with you. Exercise is also much less intimidating when you have someone to give you proper instruction.

If you choose to consult with a doctor about your weight-training or aerobics program, it should be someone with a sports medicine or physical therapy background who can help you devise a program attuned to your strength and ability. Begin by having your doctor or physical therapist show you a simple exercise, the standing biceps curl, for example. (This and other exercises will be discussed later.) Start with a very light weight to warm up, then have your doctor increase the weight to one that is much more difficult for you to lift. The entire first session should take roughly 10 minutes.

Generally, it will take you anywhere from three to six visits to a doctor or physical therapist before you can do the exercises on your own, perhaps longer if you are a novice. When you have reached a point when you can exercise on your own, correct form and movement should be almost automatic for you. It is always a good idea to occasionally have a refresher session with your doctor, especially if you change your program dramatically.

Another option for learning proper form when beginning weight training is to meet with a qualified personal trainer. Personal trainers come in many varieties—some come from body-building backgrounds, some are would-be actors, some ex-jocks; some have superb credentials, others little to none. The very best endorsement for a personal trainer is certification from the American College of Sports Medicine, which is widely regarded as the "gold standard" of personal-training certification. Even more important, you should get personal recommendations from at least three to four people whom they have trained. Also, never buy into a plan of future training sessions. Pay as you go until you have built a comfortable relationship with the trainer. Some physical therapists and medical doctors have lists of quality trainers whom they can recommend to you. Again, attend several sessions until you are comfortable doing the exercises on your own.

Method 2: Join a Gym

I usually recommend that my patients join a gym whenever possible—especially when starting—rather than buy exercise equipment for home use. Studies have shown that people tend to exercise more and comply better, and more consistently, with a program when they work out at a gym instead of at home.

Many gyms will offer you a short trial membership, usually about two weeks, or free initial sessions with a personal trainer. Going to a gym full of motivated people exercising combined with the assistance of a personal trainer can make it much easier to motivate yourself to stick with the program.

Method 3: Find a Training Buddy

Dragging yourself to the gym for the first time can be very challenging, and it provokes fear in many of my patients. One way to combat these feelings is to find a training buddy. You and your buddy can help stimulate and motivate each other as well as share the responsibility of actually getting to the gym to work out. You also may be able to save money on a personal trainer if you and your buddy schedule a joint session.

HORMONALLY CHARGED EXERCISE

Exercise can be one of the most frustrating aspects of losing weight. Many of my patients complain to me that they have spent countless hours exercising and yet have not lost a pound of body fat or even any weight. In fact, some people even gain weight from exercising! This happens because the wrong exercise program can cause your hormones to work against you and actually trigger muscle loss and fat gain. For example, excessive aerobic exercise can actually deplete your testosterone and cause your cortisol levels to rise, leading to loss of muscle and, therefore, your fat-burning potential.

But a well-regimented, hormonally stimulating exercise program can do just the opposite: help you shed the fat from your body while you maintain, or even gain, muscle. In fact, exercise has so many healthful benefits—promoting weight loss, protecting against illness, enhancing sexual performance—that I call it one of nature's "wonder drugs." But in order to actually reap these benefits from your exercise program, you must carefully plan what type of exercise you are going to do, when you are going to do it, and at what intensity. Remember that your fat is not going to magically turn into muscle; you will have to stimulate your hormones to burn fat through cardiovascular exercise and build muscle through weight training. In this chapter, I will take you step by step though my hormonally charged workout plan.

Exercise Timing

Your body has many natural hormonal cycles during the day, making the timing of your exercise program crucial to optimally harnessing your fat-burning hormones. Just as prescription drugs have indications on what time of day they are to be taken in order to maximize their effects, your workout program needs to be planned so that the benefits of the exercise can be fully realized by your hormonal system.

Early-Morning Exercise

By far the best time to exercise is in the morning, when your testosterone levels are at their highest and insulin levels are at their lowest. By exercising when your testosterone levels are at their highest, you can be sure that you are burning calories from fat rather than muscle. The testosterone boost you get from your workout also will provide you with energy and strength for the rest of the day, a more relaxed temperament, and relief from stress. And because your insulin levels are low, you avoid insulin's tendency to trigger your body to fuel exercise with muscle burn and instead you will burn off your fat.

Another advantage of working out in the morning is that your metabolism will increase for the rest of the day. Exercise has an afterburn effect that can last as long as 12 hours. Because your metabolism slows significantly when you sleep, you will lose much of this afterburn effect if you exercise late in the evening or right before bed, and you may even have trouble sleeping, particularly if you work out after 9:00 P.M.

There are several precautions for working out early in the morning. When you first wake up, your joints can be stiff and your spinal disks can be swollen from the nighttime inactivity—a problem that increases as you age. Therefore, you should always start your morning workout with a longer warm-up than you would in the afternoon. Slow walking, light jogging, gentle stretches, and other light aerobics are ideal for warming up and getting your circulation going. After 10 to 20 minutes, you should start to feel your muscles getting slightly warmer, a sign that you are ready to move on to more intense exercises.

Do not do any extreme forward or back bends that can harm your lower back and disks, aggressive neck rolls that can be injurious to the nerves of your neck, or extreme end-range motion stretches that can put too much strain on your muscles. If you have coronary artery disease (have had or are at a high risk for a heart attack or myocardial infarction, or experience angina), it is probably not a good idea to exercise at all in the early morning as it can be irritating to the coronary blood vessels.

I realize that many people these days have tight schedules that do not allow them to exercise in the morning. Instead, these people should try to exercise as early in the day as possible, perhaps during lunch. Some of my patients even divide their exercise into two sessions, taking a brisk (sweat-inducing) half-hour walk during their lunch break and then lifting weights at a gym or at home right after work.

While it is important to try to exercise as early in the day as possible, it is even more crucial to simply find time in your schedule to work out at least every other day—even if it isn't until 6:00 or 7:00 p.m. I often advise my patients to schedule "appointments" to exercise the same way you would schedule a business meeting or a visit to the dentist.

Exercise on an Empty Stomach

There is one inflexible rule for exercise timing: work out when your stomach is empty—4 hours after your last large meal or 3 hours after a smaller meal or snack. When your stomach is empty, your insulin levels are very low. Because one of insulin's main roles is to preserve your fat mass, it causes your body to burn up carbohydrates instead of fat. If you eat a sugary candy bar before exercising, your insulin levels may go through the roof, and the higher the insulin, the harder it is to lose fat. Exercising on an empty stomach enables your body to burn fewer carbohydrates and more body fat when you exercise.

Exercising on an empty stomach will also maximize your natural release of growth hormone, an indispensable component to hormonally charged fat burning. While exercise is one of the most effective ways to stimulate the release of growth hormone, if you eat starchy carbohydrates before a workout, your insulin levels will rise, blocking its release.

If you find it too difficult to exercise on an empty stomach, you can drink one to two scoops (20 to 30 grams) of a very low-carbohydrate protein powder mixed in water before your workout. By "low carbohydrate," I mean less than 2 grams of carbohydrates per serving. These kinds of protein drinks consumed before exercise can help deliver amino acids to your muscles, thereby stimulating increased growth and ensuring that you burn fat and not muscle. Drinking coffee also can help to energize and motivate you as well as speed up your metabolism before a workout.

If you get "shaky" (hypoglycemic) during exercise, you can mix a small amount of juice that is low in sugar and not syrupy with your protein powder or some nonfat milk with your coffee. To avoid dehydration, make sure you drink plenty of water before and after exercising, especially if you are exercising outdoors on a sunny day.

Exercising early in the day and on an empty stomach whenever possible will give your exercise program the extra edge needed to burn optimum levels of fat. High testosterone and low insulin is the perfect combination to hormonally charge your workouts for maximum fat loss.

Type of Exercise

In this program, you need to find a balance between aerobics and weight training. These two main types of exercise have extremely different effects on your body and your hormones. Unlike many other programs, the Hormone Revolution program emphasizes weight training because it has powerful effects on building and preserving muscle and boosting your fat-burning hormone levels. Aerobic exercise, when done correctly, strengthens and improves the function of your heart and helps burn fat. Practiced together within the same program, these two forms of exercise fuel each other and enhance your weight-loss potential. But you have to be very careful of which aerobic and weight-training exercises you do and of the duration and intensity with which you do them.

The strong potential that aerobic exercise and weight training have to stimulate hormones causes them to have druglike effects on the body, and they should be treated as such.

Aerobic Exercise

Aerobic exercise is defined as low- to moderate-intensity exercise that works the larger muscles in your body, performed for long durations of time. The aerobic exercises most beneficial to fat-burning hormone stimulation are those that employ your bigger muscle groups, such as the quad muscles in your legs. Because you are working larger muscles, you are able to burn more fat with each movement. The two best exercises for your quads are stair climbing and hill walking, which can be done on an inclined treadmill. If these machines are too hard on your knees, I recommend the elliptical exercise machines, which work the quad muscles while being easier on your knees. In addition to harming your knees and other joints, exercises such as running and jogging are not as effective for weight loss since they tend to exercise only smaller muscle groups, such as the calves, diminishing the amount of fat burned.

Swimming and cycling, although aerobic by definition, are not effective hormone boosters or fat burners. While performing both of these exercises, your body avoids the effects of gravity, diminishing the workout for your muscles and skeletal system. Studies have shown that over time these kinds of exercises are more likely to lead to bone and muscle loss. If you have bad arthritis, a few minutes in a warm pool to warm up before exercise is okay. But in general, try to avoid swimming and cycling as your main sources of aerobic exercise.

I also strongly advise against the Pilates exercise system. This is heavily promoted by some trainers and gyms, but I have found it to be a useless fad. The horizontal exercises recommended by this system are counterproductive for the Hormone Revolution program as they don't take advantage of the effects of gravity to build muscle and strengthen bones. The movements involved in this training do not enhance any function used in our daily lives. If you are serious about the Hormone Revolution program, then you must stop exercises that are not weight bearing or are not upright, such as excessive biking or swimming.

If you do your aerobic exercises too intensively or for too long, they are no longer aerobically beneficial. Excessive aerobic exercise will put your body into a survival mode as though your life were being threatened, a state that triggers the release of stress hormones such as cortisol and lowers your testosterone levels. You will no longer be burning fat but muscle.

Some exercise machines, such as stair climbers and treadmills, can help you gauge the intensity of your workout with their heart rate monitors. Make sure you set these machines for "fat-burning" mode, which will let you know when your heart rate is at 50 to 60 percent of its capacity—the target range, depending on your fitness level, for your heart rate for aerobic exercise. If your heart rate is above this level, the machine will tell you to slow down, and if you are below, it will tell you to speed up. If you are not working out on a machine that can measure your heart rate for you, you can simply count your heart beats for one minute. The formula for figuring your maximum heart rate is 200 minus your age.

For beginners or for people who have not exercised in a long time (such as couch potatoes), I recommend starting out by doing aerobic exercise three times per week for 20 to 25 minutes per session. Every couple of weeks, you can slowly increase the frequency and length of exercise sessions, but aerobic exercise should always be done at low to moderate intensity according to your fitness level. The very maximum amount of aerobic exercise I recommend is six times per week, 60 minutes per session. Always take at least one day off a week to let your body rest and repair.

Often, when you are warmed up from lifting or doing cardio, you may not feel any pain. The true sign of overdoing it is what you feel the next day. Muscle and tendons do not ably transmit pain to your brain when they are in the middle of a good exercise session. During a workout, your brain also produces natural hormones that make you feel high and block feelings of pain. You may not feel an exercise injury unless you have done something drastic like sprain an ankle or severely pull a muscle. I most frequently see symptoms of overexertion when people have been doing the same exercise repeatedly without taking time to recover or have been using a bad technique. The answer to this problem is exercise periodization and splits (which will be discussed later in the chapter).

Weight Training

Weight training is a resistance exercise that is, by definition, the opposite of aerobics. Specifically, it is high-intensity, short-duration exercise expressly meant for building and preserving muscle mass and increasing strength. Weight training is often neglected and misunderstood by most people trying to lose weight and fat. Most dieters focus entirely on aerobic exercise, which can cause you to lose a large amount of muscle mass. This muscle may be lost forever, and the loss will ultimately inhibit you from burning excess fat. Weight training solves this problem by increasing your testosterone levels, helping you preserve and build muscle, facilitating fat burning, and stimulating muscle tissue growth. By maintaining or gaining some muscle mass, you also are able to prevent the decrease in your metabolism that occurs with most weight-loss programs.

Many women avoid weight training because of the misconception that they will get too muscular. However, for many reasons, it is exceptionally difficult for women to become very muscular by natural means. The extremely muscular female bodybuilders you sometimes see in fitness magazines generally take large doses of anabolic steroids as well as many other drugs. Some of these women also have "super genes" that give them a genetic ability to get muscular very quickly. But these women are very rare. The average woman will not get bulky muscles, especially women over the age of thirty.

High-intensity weight training means that you are using a heavy enough weight to fatigue your muscles quickly after a short number of sets and repetitions. When your muscles "fail," they usually quiver and feel worn-out to the point that you just can't lift anymore. Don't be afraid to push your muscles to this quivering failure; this is a natural reaction to healthy weight training. However, do not push yourself to the point that you feel any acute or sharp pain. Feeling some discomfort is normal, and over time you will learn to read your body and be able to distinguish between good discomfort and pain that could indicate early signs of muscle, tendon, or nerve injury.

If you are new to the weight-lifting part of the program, avoid pushing too quickly to achieve moderate- or high-intensity lifting. It is always safer to begin slower with lighter weights to make gradual progress rather than to make huge gains quickly. This is especially true if you have never done any weight training or other sports, are over the age of thirty-five, or have had some prior trauma to your spine or joints.

A fundamental principle of the Hormone Revolution weight-lifting program is that you should always exercise standing up using free weights, thereby stimulating the entire body—the muscles, nervous system, and the skeleton. Lifting free weights while standing demands coordination, balance, and resistance. Also, it has been revealed that fat cells have a "stealth effect" whereby they quietly release hormones such as leptin that preserve fat stores in the body. This preserved fat is not just a storage area—each cell is a major hormone factory that has tremendous effects on many hormone systems. But recent research has shown that multijoint exercises such as squats and dead lifts help suppress this stealth effect and promote fat burning.

The stress put on your bones during weight lifting actually strengthens them, helping to prevent osteoporosis. People who have been on improper diet and exercise programs often lose excess muscle and bone mass while gaining fat, increasing their risk of osteoporosis and hip and spine fractures. Your hips and spine need some stress from gravity and weight training to increase their strength. These standing exercises are designed to increase your functional capacities for living and to improve your ability to complete everyday tasks.

I suggest that you weight-train two or three times per week, with at least one day of rest in between weight-lifting sessions. You should try to work out a different group of muscles during each of your weekly weight-training sessions, being careful not to overwork the same muscle groups. Muscles will grow only if you give them enough time between training sessions when they are not being worked: Good sleep and post-workout relaxation is essential to give your muscles time to grow and replenish.

Before you begin your weight training, you should first do some aerobic exercise. (I will give you specific recommendations for training schedules later in this chapter.) Then begin your weight training with a warm-up set of a low weight doing 20 repetitions (or reps). If you can do more than 20 reps with this weight without undue strain, then this weight is too light for a proper warm-up. Your warm-up weight should be the maximum weight that you can lift 20 times continuously yet slowly, without interruption. The purpose of this set is to get your blood flowing and your muscles ready for much heavier weights.

After your warm-up set, rest briefly for a few minutes. Now you are ready for a heavier weight. This weight should be the maximum weight with which you can do 8 to 12 reps—called your *max* (or *plateau*) lift. If you can do more than 12 reps, increase the weight at the next training session. If you can do less than 8 reps, the weight is too heavy. You should do two sets with this weight, resting at least 3 minutes between sets. After these two sets, move on to the next muscle group exercise (see section on exercise splits below). This is more than enough exercise for your muscles; any more might actually damage them, increasing your risk of injuries and lowering your testosterone levels. Brief but intense is the key to hormonally charged weight training.

Exercise Splits

A cardinal rule about weight lifting is that you must give each body part (muscle group) at least four days of rest before exercising it again. It is dangerous to exercise your whole body, working out all muscle groups three times a week. This will only lead to muscle soreness, injuries, and suppression of your fat-burning hormones. Instead, you should divide your exercise into *splits*—exercise schedules that emphasize a different group of muscles on each of your three weight-lifting days.

In the Hormone Revolution weight-lifting program, you split the body into two main sections of large muscle groups: (1) the big leg muscles (the lower half of the body and lower abs) and (2) the upper body (chest, arms, back, and upper abs). If you have really worked your muscles intensely (to the point of fatigue), then they need at least three to four days of time for their growth period (commonly called *rest-growth period*) in order to get bigger and stronger. It is during the rest and recovery period that the benefits of the exercise stimulus are reaped.

Below are two sample splits, one for those who wish to lift weights twice a week and another for those who prefer to lift weights three times per week. The two-day split requires you to do a greater number of exercises per session. If you choose a two-day split, always take at least a two-day rest in between sessions. A three-day split obviously involves one more session per week, but it also requires you to do fewer exercises at each session. There are brief descriptions of these exercises in Appendix A, but for proper instruction you should consult a qualified physician or trainer.

Two-Day Split Exercises

DAY ONE: LOWER BODY AND LOWER ABS
1. Lunge walk squats holding weights in each hand
2. Bent-legged dead lifts
3. Reverse crunches for the lower abs

DAY TWO: UPPER BODY AND UPPER ABS

1. Dumbbell bench press
2. Traditional ab crunches
3. Lateral and forward arm raises
4. Bent-over rows

Three-Day Split Exercises

DAY ONE: LOWER BODY

1. Plain squats with dumbbells in hands
2. Lunge walk holding weights in each hand
3. Bent-legged dead lifts

DAY TWO: BACK AND ABS

1. Reverse crunches for the lower abs
2. Traditional ab crunches
3. Lateral twists
4. Bent-over dumbbell rows

DAY 3: UPPER BODY

1. Lateral and forward arm raises
2. Standing dumbbell curl
3. Bent-over dumbbell rows
4. Dumbbell bench press

Periodization of Exercising

Another way to maximize the benefits of weight training is through periodization. Periodization is a system of training whereby you continually change the exercise stimulus so that the body's fat burning and muscle building do not plateau through its natural adaptive process. Your body always wants to go into the state of equilibrium or homeostasis, but by changing exercise sequences you can keep tricking the body into achieving results. After you become confident with your exercise routine, try to vary it with one of the periodization exercises described below. The longer you have been weight training, the more you will feel comfortable varying your routine and the heft of the weights you use.

Samples of Exercise Periodization

Pyramid: Always begin with a strong warm-up set. Then, using the weight that is your max lift, do 1 or 2 reps. Every 2 or 3 reps during the rest of the 10 or 11 reps in this set, use progressively lighter weights. While gradually decreasing the weights, be sure not to use weights so light that you can do more than 10 to 12 total reps.

Reverse Pyramid: First do your warm-up set. Then, with each rep, increase the weight incrementally until you hit your max lift. While it varies based on strength and the type of exercise, men can generally increase the weight by 5 pounds after each set, and women can increase by that or a smaller amount (as low as 1 or 2 pounds). When done correctly, you should go into muscle-lifting failure.

Machines: While I usually recommend free weights for weight training, you occasionally may want to switch to various weight-lifting machines that use pulleys to give your muscles a slightly different range of motion for your exercises and help increase muscle definition. If you are recovering from an injury, the muscle isolation provided by using machines can help you work toward eventually using free weights again. But remember that standing free-weight exercises are intended to be the core mode of exercise in the Hormone Revolution Exercise Plan because they enhance fat burning.

Weight training plus aerobic periodization: Begin by doing a good lower-body split-weight session to burn all the carbohydrates (muscle glycogen) stored in your large leg muscles. Then, do light- to moderate-intensity aerobic exercise using a treadmill or stair climber; this will specifically target your fat stores since you have burned off all your carbohydrate stores during weight training. During this periodization, it is particularly important that you don't work out too long (over an hour) or too intensely since you may end up burning muscle for fuel instead of fat. To guard against muscle burning, it is a good idea to drink a low-carbohydrate protein shake before this kind of workout. For many people, this combination of aerobic and weight-training exercise works best to burn fat faster.

SAMPLE EXERCISE SCHEDULES: WEIGHT TRAINING VERSUS CARDIO-AEROBIC

In general, it is ideal if you can concentrate on weight training (muscle building) one day and cardio (fat burning) on another so that you don't exhaust yourself and create an imbalance among your hormones. Because each of these forms of exercise works differently within your body and hormone systems, it is important to allow time for your body to respond to them independently.

On days when you weight-train, I recommend only a brief 5-to-10-minute aerobic workout to warm up and get your blood pumping. But no more aerobics than that! Below are some sample exercise plans that implement the exercise splits described above. You will notice that getting a good workout does not require impossible amounts of hours at the gym, just regularly scheduled, relatively short intervals. Remember that my preferred aerobic exercises are walking on an incline (as on a treadmill), stair climbing, or using an elliptical trainer (which is easy on the knees and back). Other healthy alternatives are brisk walking and light jogging.

Plan I: Exercising Four Days per Week

MONDAY

5 to 10 minutes of light aerobic exercise for a warm-up

Upper-body exercises (see two-day split)

Total time: 30 to 45 minutes

TUESDAY

Rest day

Rest means taking a break from formal exercise but maintaining your normal daily physical routines and activities such as taking leisurely walks or climbing the stairs instead of taking the elevator. By rest, I do not mean staying in bed doing nothing but watch TV or sitting in front of your computer for hours.

WEDNESDAY

45 minutes of aerobic exercise

THURSDAY

5 to 10 minutes of light aerobic exercise

Lower-body exercises (see two-day split)

Total time: 30 to 45 minutes

FRIDAY

Rest day

SATURDAY

45 minutes of aerobic exercise

SUNDAY

Rest day

Plan II: Exercising Six Days per Week

MONDAY

5 to 10 minutes of light aerobic exercise

Upper-body exercises (see three-day split)

Total time: 30 to 45 minutes

TUESDAY

45 minutes of aerobic exercise

WEDNESDAY

5 to 10 minutes of light aerobic exercise

Ab and back exercises (see three-day split)

Total time: 30 to 45 minutes

THURSDAY

Rest day

FRIDAY

45 minutes of aerobic exercise

SATURDAY

5 to 10 minutes of light aerobic exercise

Lower-body exercises (see three-day split)

Total time: 30 to 45 minutes

SUNDAY

45 minutes of aerobic exercise

Modifications to Exercise Plans

1. The first week or two that you are following the program, you might want to start out with 15 to 20 minutes of aerobic exercise and slowly work your way up to 45 minutes.

2. Remember that you can count brisk walking, such as walking your dog, as aerobic exercise. This can help you fit the aerobic portion of your exercise into your schedule.

3. If you have a week that is especially busy, such as a deadline at work or a final exam, there are ways to work around this. But try to avoid cutting out your weight-training exercise that week, and instead scale back your aerobic exercise. It is important to keep working out your muscles while you are on the program. However, if you are on a three-day split for weight lifting, during busy weeks you can revert to lifting weights only twice a week to save time.

"NON-EXERCISE" EXERCISE

There are several simple ways you can improve your overall fitness and work some "hidden" exercise into your program, especially on your days in between workouts or when you are too busy to get to the gym.

- Take the stairs whenever possible. Don't waste your time waiting for an elevator.
- Don't circle the block several times to find parking. Instead, park a few blocks away on purpose and get in a little bit of extra walking.
- Instead of going out to eat during your one-hour lunch break at work, pack your lunch and go on a 20- to 30-minute walk after you eat. Motivate some of your coworkers to do this with you in an effort to get in better shape and lose weight and fat.

- Drink lots and lots of ice-cold water. This doesn't sound like hard exercise, but your body burns up calories reheating your body every time you cool it down with ice-cold water. Most people do not drink enough water anyway, so this is a healthy practice in general.

While these activities are not especially exhausting, they can make a difference in your program. You can easily lose an extra 1 to 2 pounds of body fat per month by taking these simple steps.

THREE

THE HORMONE REVOLUTION
EATING PLAN

BEGINNING YOUR DIET

Far too many people start their diets with a "bang" by rapidly losing several pounds, only to quickly crash and end up binge eating and regaining all the weight they lost—and then some. To avoid this, you should think of your diet as a journey to weight loss. You are traveling from your current state of being overweight to your new destination of a lean, fit, and healthy body. But you need to navigate carefully to get to your new destination. Drive in the wrong direction and you will never reach your goal; drive too fast and recklessly and you will crash. This chapter will tell you how to move your weight-loss program in the right direction through recipe planning, shopping, eating, and monitoring your diet. You also will learn how to navigate your way through the many obstacles, such as dietary imbalance and overindulgence, you might face on your road to permanent weight and fat loss.

Getting Started

For your first week on the Hormone Revolution program, do not change your eating habits. You heard me right—eat exactly what you were eating before you decided to start my program. I believe that changing your habits has to come slowly, one step at a time; if you try to change everything too quickly, you will be less likely to adhere to any new system. Therefore, for the first week on the Hormone Revolution program, start exercising exactly as I have outlined to develop some strength and build an exercise foundation.

The eating plan in this program is specifically designed to hormonally charge your exercise program. During the end of the second week of exercising, slowly start to change your eating habits in order to bring them in line with the goals of the diet program outlined below:

- Regulate your dietary sources of carbohydrates based on their fiber content—the higher, the better.
- Limit your starch and sugar intake to the Magic Window period (see page 42) after exercising.
- Eliminate junk foods in favor of four to six low-starch, high-protein Standard Meals throughout the day (see page 64 and the recipes that follow).
- Coordinate your eating habits with your Hormone Revolution Exercise Plan.

Each of these elements has a tremendous impact on your hormones, as you will learn throughout this chapter. By the fourth week of the diet, you should be adhering very closely to the guidelines of the eating plan.

You will be surprised how painless this diet can be if you implement it slowly and start exercising and strengthening your body first. What do you think your body wants you to feed it after doing an intense 45-minute weight-lifting workout? A bag of potato chips or some grilled fish with rice? Research studies as well as my own observations have shown that people almost automatically start eating healthier once they begin exercising. When you exercise regularly, your body sends strong messages to your appetite and taste centers telling them what kind of food it needs, and most people respond positively to these brain messages.

CARBOHYDRATE TIMING
AND THE "MAGIC WINDOW"

Are All Carbohydrates Bad?

Low-carbohydrate diets have become the latest health fad. It seems strange that just a few years ago grocery stores were full of low-fat diet products: low-fat ice cream, cookies, even potato chips. Of course, nobody lost any weight by consuming these products. But a lot of people had a good time pigging out on all of this low-fat junk food, thinking that it wouldn't make them gain weight.

Now that people have caught on that low-fat diets don't work, they are switching in droves to low-carbohydrate diets. Led by books highlighting programs such as the Atkins diet, the Zone diet, the Protein Power diet, the Sugar Busters diet, and many others, people are racing to jump on the low-carb bandwagon. Now, instead of stocking primarily low-fat products, grocery stores and health food stores are full of low-carb food products: cookies, chocolate bars, even pancake mixes. One fad quickly replaces another.

It is true that by avoiding carbohydrates, you can lower your caloric intake. But in the long run, completely neglecting carbohydrates will ultimately be counterproductive. If you exercise regularly, carbohydrates will initially be stored not as fat but as fuel in your muscles to give you the energy for your workouts. A lack of carbohydrates may actually lead to injuries and loss of muscle. Therefore, any successful weight-loss program must allow your body the necessary carbohydrates to feed and replenish your muscles after exercise.

When the low-carb craze began, the medical community was quick to condemn it. The American Heart Association has just issued a statement condemning low-carbohydrate diets as hazardous to your health because they potentially promote heart disease. Other doctors have warned of risk of kidney problems, high cholesterol, bone loss, and many other undesirable conditions. These cautions are all in addition to the AHA's more general criticism that low-carb diets simply do not work.

While I agree that complete restriction of carbohydrates is not an effective way to lose weight, I find these claims by the medical community to be an oversimplification of the case. The high protein content of many low-carb diets is unhealthy for people with kidney problems but not for the general population. While there is a possibility that the high fat content of some diets may increase cholesterol levels, people can avoid this if they eat healthy fats such as olive oil, canola oil, or fish oil; only saturated fats such as those found in meat are linked to higher cholesterol levels. And while bone loss is a concern for older people who eat large amounts of protein, it can be prevented by taking extra calcium or vitamin D supplements and by exercising. So not all alternatives to carbohydrates are bad ideas.

But are carbohydrates as super-fattening as the proponents of low-carbohydrate diets claim? Again, the truth is not so simple. The answer lies in both *when* you eat carbohydrates and the *type* you eat. Some carbohydrate foods, like those high in fiber, are not fattening at all, regardless of when you eat them. Even those that are fattening can still be eaten if you do it at the right time—for example, after you exercise. As with all things in the Hormone Revolution program, by applying a method that takes your hormones into account, you can regulate how your body reacts to a certain stimulus. Rather than simply eliminating carbohydrates from your diet, instead you can plan meals that contain high-quality types of carbohydrates to be eaten at a hormonally beneficial time—the best time being the Magic Window.

The Magic Window

All of the low-carbohydrate diets caution you strongly against eating starchy carbohydrates such as white bread, white rice, or pasta. If eaten at the wrong time or in excess, these carbohydrates will increase your insulin levels, causing your body to store fat very quickly, increase your appetite, decrease your metabolism, and even promote muscle loss. However, you can bypass the negative effects of insulin if you eat these starchy carbohydrates at the right time. In fact, they can actually help your diet if you correctly time your consumption of them.

Exercising for 30 minutes or longer creates a climate in your body that I call the *Magic Window,* a time when your body will actually use carbohydrates to generate muscle growth. While you are working out (especially while weight lifting), you are depleting the carbohydrates in your muscles. After your workout, carbohydrates, especially starchy ones, are the prime fuel that your muscles crave to allow them to repair and recover. It is through this recovery process that your muscles actually grow. During the Magic Window, which lasts for roughly 30 to 60 minutes after exercising, you won't experience the increase in appetite or high insulin levels that you would normally get from starchy carbohydrates.

Keep in mind that you need to earn the Magic Window. A quick 10-minute workout won't cut it: Exercise too little or not intensely enough and you won't have a Magic Window. You need to follow the exercise plan outlined in the previous chapter in order to actually trigger the effects of the Magic Window.

One of the most common complaints from people who have been on the Atkins diet or other severely restrictive low-carb diets is that they crave starch. But, by using the exercise-induced Magic Window, you are able to satisfy your carbohydrate cravings without the fattening effects. Getting lean and fit does not have to mean giving up your favorite foods, just carefully timing when you eat them.

Carbohydrate Types

When you are not in the Magic Window, you need to pay very close attention to the types of carbohydrates you are eating. Many diets, including the

Zone, regulate carbohydrate intake based on the glycemic index, which is a measure of how quickly carbohydrates enter your bloodstream as sugar. As we learned in Chapter 1, overstimulation of insulin due to excessive carbohydrate intake leads to fat storage. But I find diets that heavily emphasize this fact misleading, as carrots end up having a high glycemic index (meaning they strongly provoke insulin activity), whereas pasta has a low glycemic index. Yet I am sure that nearly every doctor and dietitian will agree that carrots are much less fattening than pasta!

Therefore, to determine more accurately which carbohydrates you should include in your diet, I categorize them based on their fiber content instead their glycemic index rating. Fiber is technically classified as a carbohydrate, but it is far different from other carbohydrates in several important ways. One major difference is that fiber has zero calories. In fact, since chewing and digesting it actually burn calories while you eat, fiber is often classified as having negative calories.

Fiber also can be a strong appetite suppressant. The bulk that fiber provides in your stomach is a signal to your brain that you have eaten enough, allowing you to get full without calories. The amount of chewing required when eating high-fiber foods such as crunchy vegetables also signals your brain to turn down your appetite.

Fiber also slows down your digestion and delays the absorption and breakdown of starchy carbohydrates. Fiber coats and protects starchy carbohydrates, making it more difficult for your digestive enzymes to reach them. As a result, carbohydrates are digested more slowly, which means that your blood sugar levels will not increase as much when you include high-fiber vegetables in your meals. The combination of the slower emptying of your stomach and lower blood sugar levels will signal your appetite-regulating hormones to make you feel fuller and more satisfied.

In order to take advantage of the appetite-regulating benefits of fiber, I recommend eating at least 30 grams of fiber a day, with each meal (except the Magic Window Meal) containing 5 to 10 grams. You will learn in this chapter how to implement foods with varying levels of fiber content—high, moderate, and low (Magic Window only)—into your meals at the time of day that maximizes their benefits.

High-Fiber Carbohydrate Sources

You can eat almost unlimited quantities of foods that are high in fiber and should attempt to include them in all of your meals, except the Magic Window Meal. Vegetables such as celery, green peppers, cabbage, broccoli, and lettuce are so high in fiber and low in calories that you can eat as much of them as you want (for a comprehensive list of foods of various fiber contents, see Table 3.1). One leaf of lettuce only has 1 or 2 calories! The only thing you have to worry about from too much high-fiber vegetables is possible stomach distress.

Moderate-Fiber Foods

This category of carbohydrate sources includes foods that do have significant amounts of fiber but cannot be eaten in unlimited quantities. Examples of moderate-fiber foods are whole-grain breads, bananas, peaches, corn, and carrots. While these foods are generally healthy and not especially fattening, they still contain a fair amount of calories and are not as filling as high-fiber foods. A slice of wheat bread, depending on the brand, can have 50 to 100 calories and a peach or carrot about 50. While this may not seem like much, it can add up after a while. Therefore, you should limit your consumption of them to one to two servings per meal, or five servings a day.

Low-Fiber Foods—Magic Window Only!

Magic Window carbohydrates are generally the "white" foods—white bread, pasta, and sugar—that are high in calories but have little or no fiber content. As explained extensively in Chapter 1, low- and zero-fiber carbohydrates don't signal the release of CCK to indicate to your brain that you are full.

Table 3.1: Sources of Carbohydrates

HIGH FIBER (SERVING SIZE UNLIMITED FOR ALL HIGH-FIBER FOODS.)	MODERATE FIBER	SERVING SIZE (ONE SERVING HAS 60 CALORIES.)	LOW FIBER (MAGIC WINDOW ONLY)	SERVING SIZE (ONE SERVING HAS 60 CALORIES.)
Artichokes	**Grains:**		Fruit juice	$1/2$ cup
Asparagus	Brown rice	$1/3$ cup	Rice cakes	2
Bean sprouts	Steel-cut oatmeal	$1/2$ cup	White bread	1 slice
Bell peppers	Whole-rye bread	1 slice	White-flour bagel	$1/4$
Broccoli	Whole-wheat bread	1 slice	White-flour pasta	$1/2$ cup
Cabbage			White rice	$1/3$ cup
Celery	**Fruits:**			
Cucumbers	Apples	1		
Eggplant	Apricots	4		
Garlic	Blackberries	1 cup		
Green beans	Blueberries	$3/4$ cup		
Lettuce	Boysenberries	1 cup		
Onions	Cherries	15		
Radishes	Grapefruit	$1/2$		
Snow peas	Kiwis	$1 1/2$		
Spinach	Oranges	1		
Squash	Peaches	$1 1/2$		
	Pineapples	$3/4$ cup		
	Raspberries	1 cup		
	Strawberries	1 cup		
	Vegetables:			
	Beans	$3/4$ cup		
	Carrots	3		
	Chickpeas	$1/3$ cup		
	Corn	$1/2$–$3/4$ cup		
	Popcorn (unbuttered)	5 cups		

Therefore, these foods can actually increase your appetite and make you hungry more often.

But this lack of fiber is actually beneficial for postworkout Magic Window meals since the high-carbohydrate content in the foods will increase insulin activity, which will replenish the fuel in your muscle cells very quickly to aid in muscle building and recovery. However, if eaten when you haven't exercised, your insulin system will store the carbohydrates as fat.

While most fruit belongs in the moderate-fiber category, fruit juice generally has zero fiber and is loaded with simple sugars, making it a Magic Window–only carb. If you enjoy the sweetness and taste of fruit, eat the whole fruit rather than just drinking the juice; it is much more filling and gives you the benefits of fiber.

For those who crave starches or sweets, the Magic Window can be a strong motivation to exercise. In the Hormone Revolution Eating Plan, you have to earn each serving of sugars or starches that you eat—but at least you can still eat them! Women can eat one serving of these foods for every 20 minutes of exercise, and men can eat one serving for every 15 minutes of exercise. This doesn't mean you should exercise for 3 hours straight so you can pig out at Dunkin' Donuts. Limit your daily exercise to 1 hour, which means you can eat a maximum of four servings of low-fiber carbohydrates per day for men and three servings for women. Most important, remember that you have to eat them within 30 to 60 minutes of exercising.

Best of Both Worlds

Dieting no longer means giving up your favorite starchy carbohydrates. You can literally have your cake and eat it too—provided you eat it after working out. By using the Magic Window, your chances of long-term successful weight loss are far greater. First, it is much easier to stick to this diet because you can eat your favorite pastas or sweets once a day as long as you use the Magic Window. Thus, you won't feel deprived and won't be tempted to give up your diet. Also, you will be keeping your muscles full of carbohydrate fuel from your postworkout Magic Window Meals. This is important for maintaining strength and energy during workouts and for preserving muscles. Most low-carbohydrate diets will deplete your muscles of carbohydrates and lead to loss of muscle mass. And, most important, by paying attention to the type and timing of your carbohydrate intake, you will be maximizing the power of your hormones.

FATS AND PROTEIN: THE RIGHT TYPES AND PROPORTIONS

Like carbohydrates, different types of fats and proteins also have profound effects on your hormones contingent on the proportions you eat and when you eat them (especially in relation to exercise). It is also important to eat a proper balance of protein, carbohydrates, and fat because each of these sources of calories affects your hormones in vastly different ways. If you've read a lot of diet books, you are probably used to implementing some precise ratios of carbohydrates/protein/fat, such as 40/30/30 or 50/25/25, into your diet. But, oftentimes, when people adhere to strict ratios, they obsessively begin counting calories, losing track of what should be a vital goal of any diet—finding the best, most healthful food sources.

There is no magic ratio of calorie sources that will lead you to a fantasy world of easy weight loss, as some authors suggest. Instead, knowing how and when to integrate the proper kinds of fats and proteins into your diet, along with the carbohydrate recommendations already discussed, will allow for a hormonal response that will further your weight-loss program. If you completely eliminate fat from your diet, your body will sense starvation and will lower your testosterone levels and boost cortisol as a survival mechanism. Eating some healthy fats, such as monounsaturated fats, will help keep you in reproductive mode and thus help you maintain higher testosterone levels.

Fats

Healthy Fats

When diets such as the Atkins diet became popular by allowing you to eat almost unlimited amounts of fat, provided you avoid carbohydrates, the American Heart Association condemned them as hazardous to your health for reasons similar to those supporting their misguided view on carbohydrates. Both of these perspectives, however, fail to take into account, and distinguish between, the different types of fat. Whereas some types greatly increase your cholesterol as well as your chances of heart disease, other types can actually dramatically lower your risk of heart disease and help you lose weight as well.

To most people, the concept of "good fat" is an oxymoron or an idea that is too good to be true. But many cultures have been taking advantage of the health benefits of good fats for centuries. For example, the fat content in the typical diet of people in Mediterranean countries is about 40 percent of their total caloric intake. While the typical American diet has a similar amount of fat, the source of it is harmful trans-fatty acids. But in Mediterranean countries, the main source of this fat is from olive oil, which poses a much lower risk of heart disease and obesity than that for people in the United States.

Olive oil makes such a difference because it is very high in monounsaturated fat, which is a classic example of a good fat. Monounsaturated fats not only lower your cholesterol and your risk of heart disease but also maximize the fat-burning effects of your hormones by raising your testosterone levels and lowering your insulin levels. Monounsaturated fat also works as an effective appetite suppressant because it slows the digestion and absorption of your food much in the same way as fiber (by coating carbohydrates and delaying their absorption), which helps give your brain a strong sense of fullness and satisfaction.

Another healthy variety of fats are the *omega-3 fatty acids,* oils that are essential nutrients for your body's natural functions but that cannot be produced in your body and therefore have to be ingested. These fatty acids are used by your cells to make their surfaces more fluid and reactive. As a result, your cells will require less insulin to deliver carbohydrates to them. More efficiently operating cells in your body lead to less insulin release in your body. As a result, eating the omega-3 oils can help sustain your energy levels after eating as well as delay hunger when combined with other foods.

Unfortunately, there are not many sources of omega-3 oils. Rich sources from food include oily fish as well as shrimp, lobster, clams, oysters, and some nuts. (See Table 3.2 for a comprehensive list of fat sources.) For people who don't each much seafood or nuts, there are other options in the form of supplements. Fish oil and flaxseed oil, other rich sources of omega-3s, are available as dietary supplements in the form of capsules. (For guidance on taking these supplements, see Chapter 4.)

Later in the chapter, I will outline specific shopping suggestions to help

Table 3.2: Sources of Fat

HEALTHY FATS (INCLUDE IN YOUR DIET)		UNHEALTHY FATS (AVOID AS MUCH AS POSSIBLE)	
Monounsaturated		Saturated	**Trans-fatty Acids**
Olive oil		Beef	Most margarines
Canola oil		Pork	Partially hydrogenated oils
Almond oil		Butter	(found in potato chips and many
Avocados		Cheese	other common packaged snack foods)
		Palm oil	
Omega-3 Fatty Acids		Coconut oil	**Omega-6 Fatty Acids** (Minimize)
Oily deep-sea fish		Whole milk	Corn oil
Cold marine fish		Cream	Soybean oil
Nonfarm mackerel, sardines, salmon, cod			Sunflower oil
Clams			Safflower oil
Oysters			
Shrimp			
Brazil nuts			
Flaxseed oil			

you track down foods rich in monounsaturated fats in your grocery store as well as provide you with tasty recipes that take advantage of the hormone-balancing power of these fats.

Omega-6 Fatty Acids

Like the omega-3 fatty acids mentioned above, *omega-6 fatty acids* are essential nutrients that we can obtain only through the foods we eat. Without omega-6 fats, we are susceptible to various inflammatory and degenerative diseases such as arthritis, diabetes, and asthma. However, unlike omega-3s, overt deficiency in these fatty acids is rare. Rich sources of omega-6s include corn, sunflower, and soybean oils.

Since these oils are commonly added to many processed foods and are often found in foods that contain monounsaturated fats and omega-3s, most people get more than enough omega-6s in their diets, making it unnecessary to seek out additional sources. You should avoid cooking with oils high in omega-6 fatty acids, as they can degenerate into toxic fats when heated—another good reason to stick to oils high in omega-3s.

Unhealthy Fats

The fats that have the most potential to derail your hormonal balance are saturated fats and trans-fatty acids. These types of fats add excess calories to your diet; are closely linked to an increased risk of heart disease, diabetes, cancer, and other degenerative diseases; and can actually speed up the aging process. Saturated fats are found in most meats and dairy products: Beef, pork, butter, and cheese are some of the most common sources. Trans-fatty acids are not natural fats but are artificially manufactured and processed. You will find them in most margarines and in the oils of packaged snack foods. Unlike omega-3 fatty acids, unhealthy fats will make the surface of your cells more rigid. As a result, your cells will need more fat-storing insulin to deliver carbohydrates to them.

Many people substitute processed margarine for natural butter, but studies have shown that the synthetic trans-fatty acids found in most margarines are much worse for your health than the saturated fats in natural butter. When buying snack foods such as potato chips and packaged baked goods and donuts, check the ingredients list for "partially hydrogenated" oils, which indicates that the natural oils in the food have been altered and that the food contains trans-fatty acids. While it is extremely important to avoid saturated fats in your diet by substituting monounsaturated fats whenever possible, it is even more imperative to cut trans-fatty acids from your diet completely.

Protein

Eating adequate amounts of protein is one of the most important components of the Hormone Revolution eating plan. A diet deficient in protein can actually lead to infection, loss of immune function, starvation, and loss of muscle mass. However, a diet rich in protein has numerous muscle-building and weight-loss benefits.

Protein satisfies and suppresses your appetite much more than fats or carbohydrates by slowing down the emptying of your stomach. The structure of protein keeps your stomach full longer so that you feel satisfied for an extended period of time. If you don't believe me, try eating a slice of white bread and on another occasion half a chicken breast. Then tell me which food makes you feel more full.

Protein also speeds up your metabolism through its strong "thermic" effect, through which your body temperature rises and burns more calories. Protein speeds up your metabolism much more than fats or carbohydrates. Almost no thermic effect results from eating fat, and only a very small effect is generated by carbohydrates.

Your body also has a much more difficult time storing protein as fat than it does fats or carbohydrates, especially since fat can be stored directly without involving any chemical reactions. Protein, on the other hand, must be broken down first into sugar, which is then converted to fat, before it can be stored in this form. Each of these steps requires your body to burn calories. By the time your body has taken all these steps, it has burned almost as many calories as the protein you just ate.

Protein is also hugely important because it is the basic building block of muscle. If you exercise and reduce your calories without getting enough protein, you will just end up losing a lot of muscle. Without adequate protein, it is impossible to build or preserve muscle.

Unfortunately, many sources of protein, especially red animal meats and dairy products, are also high in saturated fats. However, there are numerous lean sources of protein that are ideal for the Hormone Revolution program. Table 3.3 below lists some good sources of high-quality protein that are also low in saturated fats.

Table 3.3: Sources of Lean Protein

Chicken breast	Tuna (in water, not oil)
Egg whites	Turkey breast
Fat-free cheese	Venison
Shrimp	Most fish and seafood
Salmon	Tempeh (fermented soy protein)

Lean sources of protein are highly satisfying to the appetite, much more so than carbohydrates, with few fattening effects. In my experience I have found that general overeating or binge eating on lean sources of protein is extremely rare. When people "pig out" or go on eating binges, it is usually on foods high in starch and saturated fats, such as pizza or donuts, never chicken breasts or tuna.

While dieting it is important to get your protein from whole foods rather than from supplements or powders. Powders containing protein sources such as whey protein are popular among bodybuilders and athletes trying to gain muscle, but they are not as filling or satisfying as real food and not recommended for people trying to lose weight. Drinking a protein shake made from water mixed with two large scoops of whey protein powder will have the same amount of protein as two chicken breasts, but it won't satisfy your appetite in nearly the same way.

The only time I advise you to include protein drinks in your diet is before a workout if you don't like to exercise on an empty stomach. An effective preworkout drink is a slow-digesting protein such as casein (a type of milk protein) or egg protein powder. Also, if you are traveling or have a very tight schedule, it may be necessary to get your protein from supplement powders or bars. While this is not ideal, it is better than resorting to fast food.

THE HORMONE REVOLUTION GROCERY CART

When you step into a grocery store, you will be tempted by thousands of different food choices, and what you choose to put in your cart ultimately determines what you put into your body. Determining which choices are the right ones is crucial to the success of your Hormone Revolution program. In this section, I will take you through the grocery store, aisle by aisle, giving you all the information you need to choose healthy foods that will maximize the fat-burning power of your hormones and help you reach your weight- and fat-loss goals.

The Breakfast Cereal Aisle

The breakfast cereal section is a dangerous part of the grocery store. Almost all breakfast cereals are extremely high in carbohydrates with little or no protein or fiber. This holds true even for cereals widely touted in natural food circles as being healthy, such as granola and muesli, both of which are very high in calories and carbohydrates. Unless you plan on using breakfast as your Magic Window Meal after exercising, most breakfast cereals should be avoided.

The exceptions are the few cereals that are actually quite high in fiber—those that have a minimum of 5 grams of fiber and less than 100 calories per serving. One brand of cereal, Fiber One, even has 13 grams of fiber per serving. Steel-cut oats, such as McCann's Irish Oatmeal, are another option for a high-fiber cereal, but make sure you avoid processed, quick-cooking oat mill, such as Quaker or McCann's instant oatmeal, which has had most of the fiber removed or broken down.

These high-fiber cereals can be very filling and will not produce a strong insulin response in your body, thus allowing your hormones to stay in a fat-burning mode. Most other low-fiber cereals are loaded with so much starch or sugar that they will push your insulin levels through the roof, making fat burning almost impossible.

The Dairy Aisle

Fortunately, the egg and dairy section of the grocery store usually provides you with a greater variety of healthy alternatives. For example, you can always find milk in at least three varieties—whole, 2 percent, and skim (nonfat)—some healthier than others. Many people often mistake the meaning of the fat percentage on milk labels, as it is a different method of fat measurement than on many nutritional labels. If you buy 2 percent milk, that actually means that 2 percent of the total weight of the milk comes from fat, not that 2 percent of the calories in the milk come from fat. In fact, one-third of the calories in 2 percent milk comes from saturated fat—an unhealthy figure. Skim milk, with 0 percent fat, is obviously a much better option.

Most grocery stores offer milk alternatives, such as soymilk, for those of you who are lactose intolerant or vegans. However, you must be careful when choosing soymilk, as most brands are loaded with sugar and carbohydrates and have very little protein. Try to choose a brand of soy milk that gets at least one-third of its calories from protein. To calculate this yourself, take the total amount of protein grams per serving shown on the label and multiply it by four. This will give you the total amount of calories coming from protein. If this number is more than one-third of the total amount of calories per serving, than this brand is a good choice. Typically the best choices of soymilk are the ones labeled "plain" or "unflavored"; the vanilla- or chocolate-flavored soymilks are usually the highest in sugar and carbohydrates. I recommend brands such as Silk, Vitasoy, and Whole Foods.

As mentioned before, margarine and butter substitutes and spreads that contain partially hydrogenated oils should be strictly avoided for their trans-fatty acid content. Healthier choices for margarine include various brands that use canola oil as a base, such as Promise or Benecol. These can help you lower your cholesterol levels and optimize your fat-burning hormones. A few companies also make "fat-free" margarine spreads. While they actually do contain a small amount of fat, it is so low that the calorie content is negligible.

Cheese is often a weak point for many people on weight-loss programs. The taste and texture of cheese are what dieters often miss the most. Unfortunately, cheese is high in saturated fat and belongs in the "indulgent food" category—foods that should be avoided except on special occasions. However, there are healthy fat-free varieties of cheese that taste and melt like regular cheese. Lifetime Specialty Cheeses offers a cheese that is made up almost entirely of milk protein and comes in many different flavors. Another alternative is feta cheese (made from goat's milk), which is lower in calories and has a more favorable blend of fats. For people who are lactose intolerant or are on a vegan diet, there are many tasty alternative cheeses made from soy or almonds, the healthiest of which derive at least one-half of their calories from protein.

Eggs are an excellent source of protein, but they are also high in fat and calories. As an alternative you can buy egg whites that come packaged in cold or frozen cartons—more convenient than removing the yolks yourself.

Despite the healthy reputation of yogurt, almost all brands are loaded with carbohydrates and sugar. Therefore, the only healthy time to consume yogurt on the Hormone Revolution Eating Plan is during your Magic Window Meal.

One of the healthiest choices in the dairy aisle is nonfat cottage cheese, which is very high in protein and low in carbohydrates and saturated fat. Low-fat cottage cheese satisfies your appetite and is a great source of high-quality milk protein.

The Meat and Seafood Counter

Whatever kind of meat and seafood you buy, it is primarily important that it is fresh. You should only shop for meat, and especially seafood, from a grocery store or market that you trust is supplied by reputable sources. Don't be afraid to inquire about the freshness of meats and where they are from.

Seafood should come from clean, nonfarmed, remote cold ocean waters; these fish feed on the extremely varied, rich natural environment, i.e., plankton, sea vegetables, and other valuable natural organisms found in the open sea. Most good seafood in the United States is flown in daily from abroad. Do not eat lake fish or any farmed fish that is caught near a large city, as it may contain unknown toxins. Farmed fish may be cheaper, but it will not contain the desired natural omega-3 oil balance. All types of fish, shrimp, crab, and even lobster are excellent sources of protein and omega-3 fatty acids, but salmon and tuna (fresh or canned in water) contain the most.

The best meat products come from animals that are raised grazing on natural grasses and plants found in clean pastures. Meat lowest in saturated fat comes from free-range chickens and lean wild game such as deer and rabbit. Generally, you should avoid red meat altogether. There are extra-lean cuts of beef, but even they are relatively high in saturated fats. If you really crave beef, you can eat one serving per week of the leanest cut of beef available. (See Table 3.4 for specific meat and seafood counter suggestions.)

Table 3.4: Meat and Seafood Grocery Cart

BUY MORE	LIMIT YOUR PURCHASES	AVOID
Skinless chicken breast	Extra-lean beef	Regular beef
Skinless turkey breast	Extra-lean pork	Regular pork
Venison	Veal	Regular veal
Rabbit	Skinless chicken parts other	Spareribs
Fish: any type, fresh or canned	than breasts	Sausage
in water (tuna, salmon, sea	Skinless turkey parts other	Chicken with skin
bass, flounder, swordfish,	than breasts	Turkey with skin
cod, etc.)		
Clams		
Oysters		
Crab		
Shrimp		
Lobster		

The Produce Section

The vegetable section gives you the most freedom in making selections for your grocery cart, as most of the offerings are high in fiber and very low in calories. In general, the most nutritious vegetables are those that are deep and rich in color: broccoli, celery, lettuce, cabbage, radishes, peppers, spinach, and many others. Starchy vegetables, such as potatoes and yams, are the only vegetables you should limit to one or two a day.

The best fruits to put in your cart are those with the highest amounts of fiber. Good choices include the berry family: blueberries, raspberries, blackberries, boysenberries, etc. You can stock up on frozen berries because they are cheap and available year-round. Most berries are good sources of fiber and low in calories. Other good choices that are low in calories and filling to the appetite include apples, oranges, and grapefruits. Try to limit your purchases of sweet fruits such as bananas, grapes, and guavas, as these fruits are high in calories and sugar.

Table 3.5: Produce-Section Grocery Cart

FRUITS		VEGETABLES	
Buy More Of (high fiber content)	Limit Your Purchases Of	Buy More Of (high fiber content)	Limit Your Purchases Of
Apples	Bananas	Artichokes	Carrots
Apricots	Cantaloupes	Asparagus	Corn
Berries (strawberries,	Cherries	Bean Sprouts	Potatoes
blueberries, raspberries,	Grapes	Bell peppers	Yams
boysenberries, etc.)	Honeydew melons	Broccoli	
Citrus fruits (lemons,	Mangos	Cabbage	
limes, oranges, grape-	Papayas	Cucumbers	
fruits, tangerines)	Pears	Eggplant	
Kiwis	Pineapple	Green beans	
Peaches	Raisins and other dried	Lettuce (non-Iceberg)	
Plums	fruits (plums, dates,	Mushrooms	
	dried berries, etc.)	Onions	
	Watermelons	Radishes	
		Snow peas	
		Spinach	
		Tomatoes	

Flavorings: Herbs, Spices, and Sauces

One of the biggest problems with the American diet is that the food is extremely bland and contains very few spices compared to the cuisines of the rest of the world. Herbs, spices, and sauces not only make your food tastier and more satisfying but also can have many health and fat-burning benefits. Some populations of the leanest people in the world are found in countries where the local native cuisine has the highest spice content. If you eat traditional hot and spicy Indian or Asian food, chances are you will eat less, thus consuming fewer calories than you would from eating bland meat-and-potato combinations typical of American cuisine.

Certain spices, especially those in the cayenne chili pepper family, create a warmer feeling that burns your taste buds, quickly stimulating your gastric juices for better absorption and digestion. Your appetite will be quenched faster, and you will actually have to eat less to feel full and satisfied. Integrating hot spices into your meals is a tasty way to reduce your caloric intake.

Certain spices even guard against the fattening effects of many foods. Garcinia cambrogia is a sour fruit native to India that gives food flavor and also blocks fat production. The ginger family of spices helps to stimulate digestion and the absorption of key minerals, which in turn helps you lose weight. Cinnamon and turmeric, among other curry powders, not only are very tasty but also have important effects on decreasing levels of insulin—the major fat-storage hormone. These spices stimulate and sensitize your cell membranes, reducing the amount of insulin they need to process sugar.

Salt adds a lot of flavor to food and is a good source of sodium (an essential mineral for our bodies), but unfortunately most Americans get too much salt in their diets from processed and canned foods. Excess can lead to high blood pressure and water retention. Fortunately, there are good salt alternatives available at most grocery stores that taste almost the same as traditional sodium-based salts. Look for salt-substitute products that contain potassium chloride, which will provide your body with potassium, the essential electrolyte mineral. Most Americans don't get enough potassium in their diets, and potassium can actually prevent the bloating created by water retention.

Sauces and salad dressings can add flavor to your food, but many are loaded with fat and add a ton of hidden calories. You should avoid sauces and salad dressings that are oil-based and instead look for those that have vinegar as their main ingredient (i.e., most fat-free salad dressings). Vinegar has almost zero calories, adds a lot of flavor to food, and has many health benefits, such as improved digestion.

If you like tomato-based sauces, such as ketchup or various pasta sauces, you might want to try making your own from fresh tomatoes instead of buying them from the supermarket. Homemade tomato sauces made from fresh tomatoes are more filling and have fewer calories than the highly processed, sugar-filled tomato sauces sold in grocery stores.

Another low-calorie sauce choice is soy sauce, but because many brands are loaded with salt, you should look for those that advertise low-sodium, which typically have only half the sodium content of regular. Teriyaki sauce is another healthy choice, as its main ingredients are soy sauce and vinegar. But be careful of brands that contain a lot of sugar—more than 3 grams of sugar per 1 tablespoon serving. Other healthy sauce choices are any that are hot and spicy, such as chili-based sauces or mustard. While these sauces have significant amounts of calories, they are so strong and spicy that only small amounts are needed to flavor your foods.

The Beverage Section

If you want to buy sweet beverages, the healthiest are those that are sugar-free and sweetened with the newly approved artificial sweetener sucralose. While sucralose has not been on the market very long, it has many advantages over NutraSweet and the other artificial sweeteners. To begin with, sucralose tastes the closest to real sugar. This isn't surprising, as sucralose is manufactured by manipulating the sugar molecule so that it has no calories. In addition, sucralose does not have the bitter aftertaste of many other artificial sweeteners and does not give people the headaches and sleep troubles that NutraSweet often does.

As mentioned before, fruit juices are generally loaded with sugars and do not have the fiber content of whole fruits. If you are thirsty, it is much more beneficial to your diet to eat a fruit—you will be surprised by how quickly your thirst disappears. Most fruits are 80 to 90 percent water and contain valuable fiber, vitamins, and minerals.

You also can make your own beverages by combining an unsweetened powder drink mix, water, and sucralose. Sucralose is now sold at most grocery stores as a powder that can be used in cooking just like sugar. You also can use it to sweeten your coffee.

The Diet and Health Food Aisle

Many "health" foods are loaded with starch and sugars, the worst offenders being "diet" shakes and rice cakes. Most diet shakes are made up of little more than sugar, a few vitamins, and a tiny amount of protein, and will not give you the nourishment you need to control your appetite. Rice cakes are highly counterproductive to your diet, as they raise insulin levels more than almost any other kind of food.

While not an ideal food, protein bars make good snacks for people who have very busy schedules or who travel a lot. Stick to the protein bars that have 30 grams of protein, less than 5 grams of sugar, and less than 300 total calories per bar. Other types of food to look for in this section are sources of friendly bacteria and enzymes that help your gut digest and absorb food. Many people overeat simply because their body doesn't properly absorb the necessary vitamins and minerals in their food and hunger returns quickly. Good sources in this section include tempeh (a fermented soy product), kefir, and natural sauerkraut.

The Bakery Section

Most baked goods should be eaten only during the Magic Window because they are usually loaded with unhealthy sugars, starches, and trans-fatty acids. Exceptions are the baked goods that are truly whole grain, containing ingredients such as whole wheat, rye, or pumpernickel, with visible whole grains. Many allegedly "whole-grain" products are about as sugar and carbohydrate laden as white bread. Make sure that white flour is not an ingredient on the label and that the only source of flour comes from whole grains. Rye products are a good choice for people with allergies to wheat, and there are even rye crackers available that are relatively low in starch and high in fiber.

The Snacks and Sweets Aisle

Most snack foods are loaded with sugars, starches, and unhealthy fats. Anyone serious about the Hormone Revolution program should avoid this section of the grocery store as much as possible. If you are really crazy about some of these foods, allow yourself to eat a few servings once or twice a week, but *only as a Magic Window food.* The only exceptions to this rule are sugar-free gelatin snacks that have only 10 calories per serving and no carbohydrates or fats. The calories come from gelatin protein, which is beneficial for repairing and rebuilding your joints and cartilage.

IMPLEMENTING THE HORMONE REVOLUTION EATING PLAN

Now that you are familiar with the best food sources of carbohydrates, fats, and proteins and with what kinds of food to buy, it is time to put this information to practical use. Specifically, you need to know how to choose and combine these foods to plan and schedule your meals to maximize the fat-burning effects of your hormones. There are two main categories of meals presented in this chapter: (1) the Magic Window Meal, which contains starchy carbohydrates or sugars, and can only be eaten right after exercise, and (2) the Standard Meal, your source of healthy proteins and fats, and high-fiber vegetables, which you should eat several times a day.

I recommend that you eat four to six times per day if at all possible—one Magic Window Meal and the rest Standard Meals. Many smaller meals throughout the day are essential to keep your blood sugar and insulin levels balanced and to avoid some of the fattening effects of insulin. You should never go longer than four hours during the day without eating in order to give your body a steady supply of nutrients and protein throughout the day to help preserve and stimulate your muscles.

But the most important reason to keep fueling your body frequently during the day is that eating the right kinds of foods will prime your body's hormones for maximum fat burning. If you go too long without eating, you can lose the fat-burning potential of your hormones. In fact, your hormones will revert to "fat storage" mode, you will lose muscle, and your metabolism will slow down.

I realize most people have busy schedules that make it difficult to eat healthy meals around the clock. This section will give you some basic advice on how to plan your daily eating habits and fit healthy foods into your tight work and social schedules.

The Standard Meal

There are two main items that should be included in every Standard Meal: a lean source of protein and high-fiber vegetables and fruits. The protein is essential for speeding up your metabolism, preserving and building muscle, and suppressing your appetite, and the fiber-filled fruits and vegetables will fill you up with little to no calories while nourishing your body. For each of your Standard Meals you should eat about 20 grams of protein (see Tables 3.6 and 3.7) and as many servings of high-fiber vegetables as you desire. An easy trick for measuring protein content is that a portion of fish, chicken

Table 3.6: The Standard Meal

ESSENTIAL		OPTIONAL ITEMS	
FOOD	SERVINGS	FOOD	SERVINGS
Lean source of protein (1 serving = 20 grams of protein)	Women: 1–1.5 servings Men: 1.5–2 servings	Moderate-fiber vegetables and fruits	No more than 5 servings a day
High-fiber vegetables	Unlimited servings	Monounsaturated fat source (canola oil, olive oil)	1 tablespoon per serving of vegetables

Table 3.7

LEAN PROTEIN SOURCE	SERVING SIZE (CONTAINS 20 GRAMS OF PROTEIN)
Chicken or turkey	3 ounces
Egg whites	5
Fish	3 ounces
Nonfat cottage cheese	⅔ cup
Nonfat cheese	¾ cup
Shrimp	3 ounces
Clams	3 ounces

Table 3.8: The Magic Window Meal

FOOD	SERVING FOR WOMEN	SERVING FOR MEN
Lean source of protein (1 serving = 20 grams of protein)	1–1.5 servings	1.5–2 servings
Starchy or sugary carbohydrates (1 serving = 15 grams of carbohydrates)	1 serving for every 20 minutes of exercise (maximum 3 servings)	1 serving for every 15 minutes of exercise (maximum 4 servings)

breast, or other lean source of protein about the size of a deck of cards contains 20 to 25 grams of protein (see Table 3.7).

If needed, you can cook your vegetables in oils high in monounsaturated fat, such as olive or canola oil. You may include a serving or two of moderate-fiber fruits or vegetables (see Table 3.1) with your Standard Meal as long as you don't exceed five servings per day. See the Hormonally Charged Recipes section later in this chapter for specific meal suggestions.

The Magic Window Meal

The Magic Window Meal is the easiest to prepare since it can be made up from a large variety of foods that many people like the best. While this is an opportunity for you to eat starchy carbohydrates, you also should include a serving of a lean source of protein. After working out, your muscles are craving both protein and carbohydrates, and by combining the two, you can boost muscle growth. Recipes for Magic Window Meals will be included later in this chapter.

Snacks

If you have been on a diet before, you have probably been told to avoid snacking. However, on the Hormone Revolution program, snacking is an essential means of implementing the four to six small meals suggested for the diet. Because most people do not have the time or energy to prepare six meals a day, the most practical approach is to prepare two or three relatively large meals and to eat two healthy snacks throughout the day.

Nonfat milk products, such as nonfat milk, cottage cheese (both of which can be mixed with berries for a snack), cream cheese, and many other cheeses, are rich in slow-digesting protein that is excellent for preserving and building muscle. Fat-free cream cheese can be used as a spread on a slice of whole-grain toast or one-half of a whole-grain bagel for a quick snack. Spread the cream cheese generously; you want to have a relatively high ratio of protein to carbohydrates.

Other healthy snack options are the various engineered foods such as the low-sugar, low-starch protein bars that are found at health food and sports nutrition stores. Opt for bars that are high in protein (20 to 30 grams), with little to no added sugar or starch and less than 300 calories per bar. There also some protein bars specifically made for women that have about 20 grams of protein and only 200 total calories.

Dining Out

In general, it is much harder to control what you eat when you dine out at a restaurant. Preparing your meals at home gives you much better control over the types of protein, carbohydrates, and fats that you eat. It is easy to find Magic Window Meals at restaurants because most menus are full of high-starch dishes, but there is often not enough time allowed in the Window to get to a restaurant. However, it is possible to find Standard Meals acceptable to the Hormone Revolution program if you choose restaurants and food carefully.

Many ethnic cuisines offer a variety of meal choices compatible with the Hormone Revolution program. In particular, traditional Asian cuisines usually contain a large amount of fish, sea vegetables, roots, and other high-fiber vegetables that are not found in the customary American diet. The Chinese and Japanese are much healthier and leaner than Americans, and obesity is almost nonexistent in most Asian countries. The Okinawan women of southern Japan are the healthiest and longest-lived women in the world, due in no small part to their healthy diets, which are made up primarily of seafood. It is only when Asian immigrants come to the United States and start eating the "American way" that obesity rapidly develops.

Unfortunately, many Asian chefs in the United States "Americanize" their food to satisfy local tastes and as a result include greater amounts of unhealthy saturated fats and other ingredients. The *kung pao* chicken and sweet-and-sour chicken or pork found in many Chinese restaurants in America are actually higher in saturated fat than two Big Macs from McDonald's. Try to frequent Asian restaurants that have a reputation for traditional, authentic cuisine and that attract ethnic clientele.

When eating at a Chinese restaurant, choose dishes that consist of chicken, seafood, or tofu combined with vegetables. Avoid sauces that are high in fat, fried dumplings, and most noodle dishes, as they, too, are loaded with starchy carbohydrates and fat. You also should limit the amount of white rice you eat or try to substitute brown rice if possible.

Korean, Japanese, and Mongolian barbecue restaurants are probably the healthiest choices when dining out because you have the most control over what type of food you will eat and how it is prepared. In these restaurants, you can watch the chef grill (not fry) meats and vegetables you select at your table, or oftentimes you can do it yourself. A meal consisting of grilled seafood or chicken breasts (not beef) with loads of fresh, colorful (and high-fiber) vegetables marinated in a tasty spicy sauce is a delicious way to meet the requirements of the Standard Meal.

As I mentioned before, the Mediterranean diet is very healthy both for staying lean and for lowering cholesterol levels. Authentic French and Italian food can be extremely healthy if you order carefully. Most important when eating Italian food is to remember that there are many delicious options besides pasta (which should never be a Standard Meal) that include fish or chicken breast with vegetables or fruit. These dishes are usually relatively low in fat and are usually cooked in olive oil or another healthy oil. The most fattening part of dining out at a good French or Italian restaurant is usually not the main course but the side orders of bread or the dessert, which should be strictly avoided for Standard Meals. You also should be wary of hidden sources of saturated fat, such as oily sauces.

However, as with all meals, I recommend that you try to prepare your own food as much as possible. Limit your dining at restaurants to no more than twice per week. No matter how careful you are with the restaurants you choose and the dishes you order, you are almost always going to consume more calories at a restaurant than you would at home.

HORMONALLY CHARGED RECIPES

Cooking your own meals allows you to have greater control over what you eat and to experiment with different flavorings and spices that can enhance your overall enjoyment of food. This section presents you with a variety of sample recipes that are compatible with the Hormone Revolution Eating Plan. The easy-to-prepare Standard Meal recipes are high in lean sources of protein and fiber and low in saturated fats. With the assistance of my expert team of nutritionists, I have assembled some choices suitable for breakfast, lunch, dinner, and even snacks. Calorie and other nutritional information is included but should only be considered as rough estimates since actual calorie count can vary based on the quality of ingredients. All of these recipes are easy, quick, and delicious!

Breakfast Choices

If you choose to make breakfast your Magic Window Meal after a morning workout, you have many options. Most traditional breakfasts are high in both starch and protein. Try to eliminate or greatly limit all sources of saturated fats from your breakfast, such as pork bacon, high-fat beef or pork sausages, butter, or whole eggs. A few Magic Window suggestions for breakfast:

- Corn flakes with skim milk and four scrambled egg whites
- Two pieces of toast with low-fat canola oil margarine and four slices of low-fat bacon alternative (turkey bacon, for example)
- French toast made with egg whites/whole egg mixture (one whole egg for every three egg whites)

The following recipes for Standard Meal breakfasts contain traditional breakfast ingredients, including eggs and fruit, which promote digestion and absorption when you first wake up while also providing you with plenty of protein for extra energy to fire up your day. Never skip breakfast.

BREAKFAST OMELET

CATEGORY: BREAKFAST

SERVINGS: 2

PREPARATION TIME: 15 MINUTES

COOKING TIME: 10 MINUTES

⅓ cup chopped onion and bell peppers

⅓ cup sliced mushrooms

1 tablespoon olive oil

1 teaspoon garlic powder

1 teaspoon sweet basil

¼ teaspoon allspice

1 teaspoon curry powder

¼ teaspoon tarragon

⅓ cup free-range turkey bacon

    (cut strips into smaller pieces as desired)

1 whole egg

3 egg whites

1 tablespoon low-fat milk

- Sauté vegetables with olive oil in a medium-size nonstick skillet over medium heat until softened.
- Add spices and turkey bacon.
- In a small bowl, beat eggs together with milk and pour over vegetable-bacon mixture.
- Cook undisturbed for 5 seconds. Push egg mixture to the center of the pan. Tilt pan to allow the uncooked eggs to run to the edge of the pan. Flip omelet and cook for another 2 minutes. Divide in half and serve immediately.

Calories	225
Protein	30 g
Carbohydrates	5 g
Total Fat	6 g
Dietary Fiber	3.8 g

Recipe courtesy of Anna Brantman.

Note: You can modify almost any omelet recipe by substituting egg whites for whole eggs. You also can add your favorite fat-free cheese to any omelet. This will add both the tasty flavor of cheese and some extra protein to your omelet. Also feel free to experiment with different vegetables in your omelet. Just avoid using pork bacon or regular high-fat cheese. Of course, avoid starchy side dishes such as potatoes and pancakes unless you are using breakfast as your Magic Window Meal.

FRUIT SALAD WITH SHRIMP

CATEGORY: BREAKFAST

SERVINGS: 4

PREPARATION TIME: 10 MINUTES

2 tablespoons freshly squeezed orange juice

2 tablespoons balsamic vinegar

1 tablespoon Dijon mustard

1 teaspoon raw honey

⅛ teaspoon pepper

2 cups cooked salad shrimp

1 navel orange, peeled and cut into ¼-inch slices, halved

2 cups sliced strawberries

Baby lettuce leaves

- Combine orange juice, vinegar, mustard, honey, and pepper in a jar with a tight-fitting lid. Cover and shake well until completely mixed.
- Mix shrimp and dressing in a bowl.
- Add the orange and strawberry slices; toss gently.
- Dish salad on baby lettuce leaves and serve.

NUTRITIONAL INFORMATION PER SERVING:

Calories	115
Protein	16 g
Carbohydrates	24 g
Total Fat	0.8 g
Cholesterol	62 mg
Sodium	129 mg
Dietary Fiber	3.8 g

Recipe courtesy of Anna Brantman.

HIGH-PROTEIN BLUEBERRY PANCAKES

CATEGORY: BREAKFAST

SERVINGS: 2

PREPARATION TIME: 5 MINUTES

COOKING TIME: 5 MINUTES

1 cup soy flour, low-carbohydrate flour,* or soy protein powder

½ cup egg whites

1 teaspoon baking powder

½ cup water

2 teaspoons canola oil

½ cup blueberries

Several companies make low-carbohydrate/high-protein baking flours, including Ketagenis Inc., Low Carb Success, and Carbolite. They are widely available at health food stores and at Netrition.com.

- Combine all the ingredients in a bowl and stir until all the lumps are gone.
- With a spoon, pour small amounts of the batter onto a lightly greased (with canola oil spray) hot nonstick pan. Add batter until pancakes reach the desired size.
- Cook pancakes until the cooked side is golden brown.
- Flip pancakes, cook until both sides are golden brown.
- Top with blueberries, low-calorie margarine (canola oil–based), or a little reduced-calorie syrup.

NUTRITIONAL INFORMATION PER SERVING:

Calories	375
Protein	43 g
Carbohydrates	24 g
Total Fat	11 g
Dietary Fiber	7 g

Note: For a whole-egg flavor, you can substitute 2 whole eggs for the egg whites and canola oil. This substitution will be tastier to some but won't be as "heart friendly." Try to find syrups with 35 or fewer calories per serving.

Lunch/Dinner Suggestions

Seafood

The following seafood recipes can be used for Standard Meal lunches or dinners. Everything from thin fillets to oysters on the half shell to large whole fish can be baked with little or no added fat required. Smaller fillets or fish pieces should cook at a high temperature (425 degrees Fahrenheit) so they can cook quickly and retain their moisture. Large pieces and whole fish should be cooked at a moderate temperature (about 350 degrees) so the heat can penetrate the interior without overcooking the exterior. Because oven heat is dry heat, it can remove moisture from seafood. Some ways to help maintain moisture are coating the seafood with seasoned bread crumbs or a brush of olive oil, topping with thinly sliced vegetables, or cooking in foil or special wrappings that prevent loss of natural juices and moisture. General baking instructions for most of these recipes are:

1. Preheat the oven. Arrange the seafood in an even layer on a lightly oiled baking dish, folding thin fish ends under for even cooking.
2. Sprinkle any seasonings or coatings called for in the recipe over the seafood.
3. Bake the seafood until it is opaque through the thickest part. The time will vary, but 10 minutes per inch of thickness is a good rule of thumb.
4. Transfer the seafood and vegetables to individual plates. Spoon any remaining cooking juices over the seafood and serve immediately.

Seared Ahi Tuna—
An Extra Protein Booster

CATEGORY: LUNCH/DINNER

SERVINGS: 2

PREPARATION AND COOKING TIME: 10 MINUTES

This is one of the most popular dishes among my patients.

3 ounces ahi tuna

Canola oil spray

Chopped garlic onions to taste

Salt and pepper or other spices to taste

- Place ahi tuna on a nonstick cooking pan that is lightly coated with canola oil spray.
- Add chopped garlic onions, salt, pepper, or other spices to taste.
- Cook over medium-high heat until the fish turns white on one side (about 2 minutes), then flip it over to the other side and cook another 2 minutes.
- When you cut into the tuna, the center will be red. Eat it alone or with a salad.

NUTRITIONAL INFORMATION PER SERVING:

Calories	150
Protein	25 g
Carbohydrates	8 g
Total Fat	1 g
Dietary Fiber	4 g

Broiled Salmon with
Sesame Spinach and Beet Salad

CATEGORY: LUNCH/DINNER

SERVINGS: 2

PREPARATION TIME: 15 MINUTES

COOKING TIME: 10 MINUTES

2 salmon fillets (about 12 ounces)

Salt, pepper, and other spices (e.g., five-spice powder) to taste

1 bunch spinach (about ¾ pound)

2 medium cooked, peeled, and thinly sliced beets
  (about 10 ounces)

4 teaspoons balsamic vinegar

½ teaspoon Asian sesame oil

Garnish: plain or toasted sesame seeds

- Season salmon with salt, pepper, and five-spice powder.
- Bake until the fish becomes opaque through the thickest part, usually 10 minutes per inch of thickness.
- Remove the stems from the spinach. Stack the leaves and cut them into ⅓-inch-wide strips. In a bowl, mix spinach with the sliced beets.
- In a small bowl, stir together the vinegar and sesame oil.
- Toss spinach and beets with the vinaigrette and garnish with plain or toasted sesame seeds.
- Serve the cooked salmon on a bed of salad.

NUTRITIONAL INFORMATION PER SERVING:

Calories	262
Protein	30 g
Carbohydrates	3 g

Total Fat	<8 g
Cholesterol	0 mg
Sodium	73 mg
Dietary Fiber	1 g

Recipe courtesy of Anna Brantman.

Note: While beets do contain some iron, the amount is small. These root vegetables are an excellent source of potassium and contain some folic acid (folate). Beet greens are also edible. Compared to beets, the greens contain higher levels of beta-carotene and calcium. The alleged powers of spinach are attributed to the vegetable's abundant iron. Spinach is indeed iron-rich, but it also contains oxalic acid, which prevents most of the iron from being absorbed by the body. However, ½ cup of cooked spinach has more than a day's supply of an important antioxidant group called the carotenes. Spinach also contains vitamin C, folic acid, and dietary fiber.

GRILLED HALIBUT SALAD

CATEGORY: LUNCH/DINNER

SERVINGS: 6

PREPARATION TIME: 30 MINUTES

COOKING TIME: 10 MINUTES

1⅓ pounds halibut, cut into 1½-inch cubes

½ cup lemon juice

1 tablespoon olive oil

1½ teaspoons minced garlic

¼ teaspoon dry crumbled mint leaves

⅛ teaspoon dry crumbled oregano leaves

1 red onion, peeled and cut into chunks

4 cups chopped baby spinach or red leaf lettuce

Garnish: 1 pint cherry tomatoes

- Rinse halibut and pat dry.
- In a medium-size bowl, combine the lemon juice, olive oil, garlic, mint, and oregano. Add halibut chunks and stir to coat the fish with the marinade. Cover and chill 30 minutes in the refrigerator.
- Preheat grill or broiler.
- Drain halibut but reserve the marinade. In a small saucepan, bring the marinade to a boil and then keep it warm.
- Skewer the fish, alternating red onion chunks with the halibut. Grill or broil 4 to 5 inches from heat source, turning fish once and basting until fish is just opaque through center (cut to test), about 10 minutes.
- Serve the broiled fish with vegetables on a bed of baby spinach or red leaf lettuce. Drizzle the salad with the warm marinade and garnish with cherry tomatoes.

NUTRITIONAL INFORMATION PER SERVING:

Calories	167
Protein	23 g
Carbohydrates	8 g
Total Fat	4 g
Saturated Fat	0.7 g
Cholesterol	32 mg
Omega-3 Fatty Acid	400 mg
Sodium	78 mg

Recipe courtesy of Anna Brantman.

TRI-ORANGE ROUGHY

CATEGORY: LUNCH/DINNER

SERVINGS: 2

PREPARATION TIME: 5 MINUTES

COOKING TIME: 10–20 MINUTES

1 teaspoon orange oil

2 tablespoons nonfat mayonnaise

1 teaspoon garlic paste

3 tablespoons orange juice

½ dropper liquid stevia extract or 4 tablespoons sucralose powder

8 ounces orange roughy fillet (Substitute red snapper fillets if orange roughy is hard to find.)

Black pepper to taste

1 orange, cut into wedges

· Mix all the ingredients except the fish in a bowl.
· Spread the mixture over the fillet.
· Broil or bake (see page 74).
· Sprinkle with black pepper to taste.
· Serve with orange wedges.

NUTRITIONAL INFORMATION PER SERVING:

Calories	140
Protein	23 g
Carbohydrates	2 g
Total Fat	4 g

Recipe courtesy of Mason Panetti.

LIME SALMON

CATEGORY: LUNCH/DINNER

SERVINGS: 2

PREPARATION TIME: 5 MINUTES

COOKING TIME: 10–20 MINUTES

8 ounces salmon fillet

Lime juice

Coarsely ground pepper

1 lime, cut into wedges

- Marinate salmon fillet overnight in lime juice.
- Sprinkle fillet with pepper before broiling for 10 to 20 minutes.
- Serve with lime wedges.

NUTRITIONAL INFORMATION PER SERVING:

Calories	233
Protein	25 g
Carbohydrates	0 g
Total Fat	14 g

Recipe courtesy of Mason Panetti.

ZESTY TOMATO FISH

CATEGORY: LUNCH/DINNER

SERVINGS: 2

PREPARATION TIME: 5 MINUTES

COOKING TIME: 10–20 MINUTES

8 ounces fillets of sole, cod, or red snapper

3 tablespoons fat-free mayonnaise

4 large tomato slices

Salt and pepper to taste

- Coat fillets with fat-free mayonnaise.
- Place slices of tomato over coated fillets.
- Add salt and pepper to taste.
- Bake as instructed on page 74.

NUTRITIONAL INFORMATION PER SERVING:

Calories	150
Protein	20 g
Carbohydrates	6 g
Total Fat	5 g

Recipe courtesy of Mason Panetti.

Note: If you do not like the "fishy" flavor of fish, you might want to substitute mahimahi (called *dorado* in Mexico) or ahi/yellowtail tuna for the fish in this and other recipes. These types of fish do not have as strong a "fishy" taste and are just as healthy.

While chicken and turkey are not as healthy as seafood, breast pieces are relatively low in saturated fat and are good sources of protein. In most of the following recipes, you can substitute turkey for chicken.

CHICKEN CURRY

CATEGORY: LUNCH/DINNER

SERVINGS: 4

PREPARATION TIME: 5 MINUTES

COOKING TIME: 25 MINUTES

1 tablespoon olive oil

1 cup finely chopped onion

3 garlic cloves, minced

1 pound skinned, boned chicken breast, cut into bite-size pieces

1 tablespoon curry powder

1 teaspoon ground marjoram

2 cups chopped tomato

1 cup fat-free, low-sodium chicken broth

½ teaspoon cayenne pepper

½ cup plain fat-free yogurt

1 teaspoon all-purpose flour

- Heat the oil in a large nonstick skillet over medium-high heat. Add onion and garlic; cook for 4 minutes, or until the onion is tender. Add the chicken and cook another 4 minutes.
- Add curry powder and marjoram and cook for 1 minute.
- Add tomato, chicken broth, and pepper; reduce heat and simmer for 15 minutes. Remove from heat.

- Combine yogurt and flour; whisk to combine. Add to chicken mixture and cook for about 1 minute, or until slightly thick.

NUTRITIONAL INFORMATION PER SERVING:

Calories	318
Total Fat	5.8 g
Saturated Fat	1 g
Protein	33.8 g
Carbohydrates	12.7 g
Cholesterol	66 mg
Sodium	225 mg

Recipe courtesy of Anna Brantman.

WATERCRESS, PEAR, AND WALNUT SALAD WITH POPPY SEED DRESSING

CATEGORY: LUNCH/DINNER

SERVINGS: 8

PREPARATION TIME: 10 MINUTES

3 tablespoons apple cider vinegar

4 teaspoons Dijon mustard

1 teaspoon raw honey

¾ cup canola oil

1 teaspoon poppy seeds

Salt and pepper to taste

2 large bunches trimmed watercress

⅔ cup chopped, toasted walnuts

2 pears, peeled and cut into ¾-inch pieces

6 ounces boned, skinned roasted chicken or turkey, cut into bite-size pieces

- Blend vinegar, mustard, and honey in a small bowl. Gradually add canola oil. Mix in poppy seeds. Season dressing with salt and pepper to taste.
- In a large bowl toss watercress with walnuts and enough dressing to coat it. Season with salt and pepper to taste. Place pears on top of the salad.
- Serve the salad with pieces of roasted chicken or turkey.

NUTRITIONAL INFORMATION PER SERVING
(INCLUDING 6 OZS. COOKED POULTRY):

Calories	163
Protein	32 g
Carbohydrates	8 g
Total Fat	2 g
Saturated Fat	<1 g
Cholesterol	63 mg

Recipe courtesy of Anna Brantman.

Note: Watercress has a cooling quality and tastes pungent and bitter. It is also a rich source of carotenes, chlorophyll, sulfur, and calcium.

GARLIC-PEPPER CHICKEN BREASTS

CATEGORY: LUNCH/DINNER

SERVING: 1

PREPARATION TIME: 10 MINUTES

COOKING TIME: 10–20 MINUTES

2 teaspoons fresh black pepper

1 teaspoon garlic powder

2 tablespoons Spike brand herbal seasoning

1 skinless chicken breast

- Preheat oven to 400 degrees Fahrenheit or preheat broiler.
- Mix spices in a small bowl.
- Spread the spices over the chicken breast and pat to adhere.
- Bake chicken for roughly 20 minutes, or broil 5 minutes on each side.

NUTRITIONAL INFORMATION PER SERVING:

Calories	140
Protein	29 g
Carbohydrates	0 g
Total Fat	1.5 g

Recipe courtesy of Mason Panetti.

LOW-CARB BREADED FRIED CHICKEN

CATEGORY: LUNCH/DINNER

SERVING: 1

PREPARATION TIME: 10 MINUTES

COOKING TIME: 10–20 MINUTES

2 cups crushed high-fiber crackers (Bran-a-Crisp or other brands)

1 teaspoon garlic powder

2 tablespoons Spike brand herbal seasoning

1 teaspoon Cajun seasoning (or more, if you prefer spicier chicken)

1 skinless chicken breast

1 lightly beaten egg white

2 tablespoons canola or olive oil

- Mix crushed crackers and spices in a bowl, then mash mixture into a powder and blend.
- Coat chicken breast with egg white.
- Put chicken breast and cracker-spice mixture in a sealed plastic bag and shake to coat.
- Heat oil in a 12-inch frying pan over medium-high heat. Add chicken and fry about 5 minutes per side, until chicken is fully cooked (no pink in the middle).

NUTRITIONAL INFORMATION PER SERVING:

Calories	390
Protein	37 g
Carbohydrates	24 g (not including fiber)
Fiber	16 g
Total Fat	13 g

Recipe courtesy of Mason Panetti.

GUILT-FREE TERIYAKI CHICKEN

CATEGORY: LUNCH/DINNER

SERVINGS: 2

PREPARATION TIME: 10 MINUTES

COOKING TIME: 10–20 MINUTES

2 tablespoons garlic paste or finely grated fresh garlic

2 tablespoons ginger paste or finely grated fresh ginger

1 cup low-sodium soy sauce

3 tablespoons Worcestershire sauce

1 dropper liquid stevia or sucralose equivalent

1 tablespoon black pepper

¼ cup finely chopped green onion

2 large chicken breasts

- Mix all ingredients except the chicken breast in a 2-inch-deep or larger baking dish.
- Pound the chicken breast until it is ½ to ¾ inch thick and place it in the baking dish with mixture, turning it to coat both sides.
- Marinate the chicken in the refrigerator for a minimum of 2 hours and up to overnight.
- Broil 5 minutes per side until done.

NUTRITIONAL INFORMATION PER SERVING:

Calories	240
Protein	31 g
Carbohydrates	5 g
Fiber	1 g
Total Fat	2 g

Recipe courtesy of Mason Panetti.

Lunch/Dinner Side Dishes

The best side dishes for Standard Meals in the Hormone Revolution Eating Plan are steamed vegetables. Broccoli, cauliflower, cabbage, Brussels sprouts, and asparagus are especially filling, low-calorie choices. You can add fat-free or low-fat margarine and spices for flavor. There is also a product called Butter Buds, which is low in calories and can be put on vegetables before steaming for a rich butter flavor.

Salads are always excellent as side dishes. The only time salads are fattening is when you load them with high-fat dressings. Stick to a tasty fat-free vinegar-based dressing, and your salad will be a satisfying low-calorie side dish for any meal. Vegetable salads are generally preferable to fruit salads, since high-quality lettuce, cabbage, and most other vegetable salad ingredients are very high in fiber and low in calories.

Other suggestions for side dishes are high-fiber unprocessed grains, barley, or brown rice. A good way to add flavor is to cook them in low-sodium, low-fat chicken broth. Garbanzo beans, a good source of protein, make an excellent side dish as well.

Magic Window Side Dishes

If you choose lunch or dinner as your Magic Window Meal, you may choose a starchy carbohydrate source as a side dish to your chicken or fish entrée. These can include white bread, white-flour pasta, potatoes, yams, or white rice. Remember to limit your servings of starchy side dishes to one serving (15 grams of carbohydrates) per 15 minutes of exercise for men and one serving per 20 minutes of exercise for women. You can even choose to have a small dessert as your Magic Window selection, provided the dessert is low in fat and meets the Magic Window carbohydrate guidelines. Serving sizes of some popular side dishes are:

- Rice cakes: 2
- White bread: 1 slice

- White-flour bagel: ¼
- White-flour pasta: ½ cup
- White rice: ⅓ cup

Snacks

Remember that snacks can make up several of your Standard Meals through-out the day and should include healthy portions of protein and fiber. The two recipes below require a minimal amount of preparation time and are easy to eat on the go. As mentioned before, other snack ideas include high-fiber fruits with low-fat cottage cheese for protein and protein bars (see the section on Snacks, page 66).

FAT-FREE CHICKEN SANDWICH

CATEGORY: SNACK

SERVING: 1

PREPARATION TIME: 5 MINUTES

3 thin slices fat-free chicken lunch meat (you can substitute turkey)
1–2 tablespoons fat-free mayonnaise (or a small amount of spicy mustard to taste)
1 slice whole-grain bread
Lettuce or other high-fiber vegetables

NUTRITIONAL INFORMATION PER SERVING:

Calories	230
Protein	20 g
Carbohydrates	20 g
Fiber	7 g
Total Fat	6 g

HIGH-POWERED PROTEIN SHAKE

CATEGORY: SNACK

SERVING: 1

PREPARATION TIME: 5 MINUTES

30 grams flavored protein powder (preferably milk or egg derived)

5 ice cubes

1 tablespoon flaxseed oil

1 teaspoon guar gum (thickening agent and fiber available in
   powdered form at most health food stores)

2 or more cups cold water

- Mix protein powder and ice cubes in a blender until ice cubes are finely crushed.
- Add flaxseed oil and guar gum.
- Add about 2 cups water (or more) until the shake reaches your desired consistency.

NUTRITIONAL INFORMATION PER SERVING:

Calories	250
Protein	30 g
Carbohydrates	1 g
Fiber	5 g
Total Fat	12 g

Note: There are many choices in brands and flavorings of protein powders, so you can experiment and find one you like. Women may wish to use only 20 grams of protein and ½ tablespoon of flaxseed oil to get a lower-calorie shake (around 150 calories). You also can add flavor and antioxidants by adding fresh berries to your shake.

Nutty Cottage Cheese

CATEGORY: SNACK

SERVING: 1

PREPARATION TIME: 1 MINUTE

1 cup low-fat (1% or 2%) cottage cheese

¼ cup slivered almonds (raw) or crushed walnuts

1 teaspoon ground flaxseeds

- Mix all three ingredients in a bowl.

NUTRITIONAL INFORMATION PER SERVING:

Calories	295
Protein	34 g
Carbohydrates	9 g
Fiber	3 g
Total Fat	15 g

Recipe courtesy of Cristiana Paul, M.S.

CATEGORY: SNACK

SERVING: 1

PREPARATION TIME: 1 MINUTE

1 cup low-fat ricotta cheese

Stevia (preferably powdered) to taste

1 tablespoon dried blueberries

1 teaspoon ground flaxseeds or slivered almonds

- Mix all ingredients in a bowl. Cover and refrigerate 1 to 2 hours to soften the dried blueberries.

NUTRITIONAL INFORMATION PER SERVING:

Calories	300
Protein	24 g
Carbohydrates	18 g
Fiber	1 g
Total Fat	12 g

Recipe courtesy of Cristiana Paul, M.S.

Other Suggestions

Remember that these recipes are just to get you started on a hormonally charged cooking path and are not meant to be a comprehensive cooking guide. Once you get started, you will be able to find additional recipes and even create your own dishes using the guidelines in this book.

One area I didn't cover very much is vegetarian cooking. This is mainly because there is a plethora of vegetarian cookbooks available at any major bookstore or health food store. If you are a vegetarian, or simply wish to prepare a vegetarian dish, keep a couple of things in mind. Many vegetarians do not get enough protein in their diets, especially those who are on an exercise program that emphasizes weight training like the Hormone Revolution Exercise Plan. To avoid this, make sure each of your vegetarian dishes has a least one good source of protein. These vegetarian sources of protein are usually soy based (such as tofu) or wheat based. Also, make sure the vegetarian dish does not contain large amounts of sugars or simple starches. Vegetarian cooking does not necessarily mean "healthy" cooking unless unprocessed vegetables, fruits, and plant proteins are used in place of sugars and starches.

Vegans (those who don't eat eggs, milk, meat, or fish) will find it the most difficult to follow the Hormone Revolution program and still obtain significant fat loss and muscle gain. It is still possible, but it will require extra diligence, study, and planning. Vegans need to be especially careful to get adequate protein in their diets.

There are many low-carbohydrate cookbooks available as well. Many of these recipes are compatible with the Standard Meal criteria of my program. The only problem I have with some of these cookbooks is that their recipes are often very high in saturated fats. Try to choose recipes from these books that are low in saturated fats, such as chicken or fish dishes. If the recipes call for high-fat sauces, try to substitute with the lower-fat alternatives suggested in the recipes in this chapter.

You will see that the Hormone Revolution Eating Plan allows for a wide variety of tasty and zesty meals. There are thousands of different ways to prepare dishes that are high in protein and low in starch and saturated fats. Use this chapter as a launching pad to begin a new hobby in cooking delicious yet tasty dishes that will help mobilize your fat-burning hormones. You will be surprised how quickly and easily the pounds and inches come off once you begin to prepare your own tasty and nutritious meals!

DAILY EATING SCHEDULES

The key factor in planning your daily eating schedule is when you choose to exercise. As mentioned before, morning is the best time to exercise, making breakfast your Magic Window Meal. As you now know, you should eat four to six small meals a day, or every 3 to 4 hours. Below in the two examples of daily eating plans, I allow for more frequent eating after quality exercise.

Example I: Exercising in the Morning

7:00 A.M. (Breakfast exercise boost):   Protein shake

7:15 A.M.:   Exercise for 45 minutes to 1 hour

8:00 A.M. (Magic Window Meal):   Five scrambled egg whites; a bowl of corn flakes with skim milk

10:00 A.M.:   Protein bar

1:00 P.M. (Lunch):   Grilled chicken salad with fat-free dressing

6:00 P.M. (Dinner):   Grilled fish or chicken breast with steamed broccoli or other high-fiber vegetable

10:00 P.M.:   Fiber crackers with fat-free cream cheese or fat-free cheese

Example II: Exercising in the Evening

8:00 A.M. (Breakfast):   Breakfast omelet

12:00 P.M. (Lunch):   Turkey breast sandwich with whole-grain bread and lettuce

5:00 P.M.:   Protein shake (30 grams of protein mixed in water)

5:15 P.M.:   Exercise for 45 minutes to 1 hour after work

6:00 P.M. (Magic Window Meal):   Grilled fish; 2 to 3 servings of white rice; 2 small oranges or 1 cup of strawberries for dessert

8:00 P.M.:   Protein bar

10:00 P.M.:   1 cup nonfat cottage cheese

Notice that in these eating plans, breakfast and dinner are the largest meals. Eating a relatively large breakfast in the morning should keep you from overeating later in the day. Dinner tends to be the time when appetites and the need for comfort are at their highest levels, so you might want to schedule a slighter larger meal at dinner than at other times during the day.

No matter how busy your schedule, there is no excuse for not having at least four meals per day. Put into your appointment book specific times to eat and exercise the same way you would schedule a business meeting or a visit to the doctor.

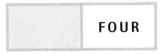

FOUR

THE HORMONE REVOLUTION
SUPPLEMENT PLAN

If you have walked into a health food or vitamin store recently, you have probably noticed the rows upon rows of shelves with all sorts of different dietary supplements. The variety and expense of most supplements can be extremely overwhelming, leaving many people to worry whether they are getting the right kind, the right amount, the best quality, or the right price. The goal of this chapter is to demystify vitamin, mineral, and herbal supplements and to show you how to integrate them into your weight-loss program.

I will present two distinct categories of supplements—the *core supplements* and the *hormone boosters* (including thermogenics)—each of which addresses specific needs that arise at different times in the Hormone Revolution Weight-Loss Plan. The core supplements should be used continuously throughout your program to compliment your diet and exercise, whereas the hormone boosters should be used only in cycles to overcome weight-loss plateaus.

While I do recommend a wide variety of supplements for different purposes, in this chapter I will focus on a few supplements that are both the most important and the most cost effective. The combination of supplements in this book will not break your bank and will generally cost about $30 to $60 per month. For more information on the other supplements I recommend, see the Supplement Resources in the back of the book.

Keep in mind that supplements are not a cure-all. They will not compensate for poor diet or lifestyle choices. However, if you are already on a solid diet and exercise plan such as the Hormone Revolution program, supplements can make a huge difference.

CORE SUPPLEMENTS

If you follow the Hormone Revolution Weight-Loss Plan closely, you will be eating a wide variety of healthy foods, such as vegetables, fruits, and lean sources of protein that will give your body many of the nutrients it needs to function optimally. Your diet, in conjunction with your Hormone Revolution cardio and weight training, will be helping you shed pounds and reap the fitness benefits of hormone balance. The next step toward achieving your weight-loss goals will be the core supplements. You should implement these supplements continuously throughout your weight-loss program.

Multivitamin and Multimineral

If you are dieting and restricting the total number of calories you are eating, the risk of a deficiency becomes even greater. Also when exercising regularly (i.e., following the Hormone Revolution Exercise Plan), your body might need extra vitamins and minerals because of increased demands on your body. Failing to get these essential vitamins and minerals could result in an increased appetite and hormonal imbalances that lead to fat storage.

The easiest way to combat these deficiencies is with a broad-spectrum multivitamin and mineral supplement. The most effective supplements that contain the widest spectrum of vitamins and minerals are those found in health food and vitamin stores rather than brands sold in grocery stores. Find a formula with at least 100 percent of the Recommended Daily Allowance (RDA) for most of the essential vitamins and minerals.

While 100 percent of the RDA of vitamins is easy to find, it is often harder to find supplements with sufficient amounts of a broad range of minerals. However, you should at least ensure that your supplement has 100 percent of the RDA of zinc, magnesium, and calcium. Zinc is especially important for this diet, as it plays an important role in regulating levels of fat-burning hormones (including testosterone) and limiting the amount of the fat storage hormone estrogen in your body. Magnesium supplementation has been shown to improve exercise performance. And calcium, especially important for people over forty, guards against bone loss and osteoporosis.

Your multivitamin should also contain ample amounts (I recommend over 100 percent of the RDA) of the antioxidant group of vitamins and minerals. Exercising can lead to some excess wear and tear on your body, but antioxidants can protect your body from this stress and can actually reduce muscle soreness resulting from exercise. The antioxidant group consists of vitamins A (in the form of beta-carotene and other mixed carotenoids), C, and E, along with the mineral selenium, a potent combination for protecting the cells in your body. These antioxidants also may help improve your immune system, protect you against various cancers, and even promote a stable balance of fat-burning hormones. To maximize these benefits, try to find a formula with at least 10,000 IU (International Units) of beta-carotene and other carotenoids, 400 IU of vitamin E (preferably the natural oil form), 500 milligrams of vitamin C, and 50 micrograms of selenium.

Multivitamin/multimineral formulas usually come in individual packets with two to four pills in each packet and should be taken with breakfast in the morning. While this may seem like a lot of pills to take, they are necessary, as it is impossible to put all the essential vitamins and minerals with extra amounts of the antioxidant group into one single pill. There also are "A.M./P.M." formulas that have an energizing vitamin/mineral combination for the morning and a sleep and relaxation formula for the evening.

Essential Fatty Acids

As you will recall from Chapter 3, the omega-3 fatty acids that are essential to your body's functioning can reduce the fattening effects of insulin and focus your hormones on fat burning rather than fat storage. Omega-3 fatty acids will stabilize your blood sugar and insulin, particularly benefiting those who are prone to hypoglycemia or diabetes. Many people notice sustained energy levels after taking an omega-3 supplement, which is largely due to its effects on blood sugar and insulin. Omega-3 fatty acids are found in most seafood and various nuts, but, unless you eat seafood every day, you will need an additional omega-3 supplement.

The most common forms of omega-3 supplements are fish oil capsules and flaxseed oil liquid. Fish oil is quite potent, and the recommended dose is usually only 2 to 4 grams per day. The typical dose of flaxseed oil is ½ to 1 tablespoon per day. Both should be taken first thing in the morning with breakfast. These oils do not keep well, so unopened supplements should be stored in a cool, dry place and, once opened, in the refrigerator. Some omega-3 supplements contain vitamin E to help preserve freshness.

HORMONE BOOSTERS

The second category of supplements consists of those that can be used to overcome weight-loss plateaus—the hormone boosters. After a few months of achieving results, many people notice a decline or full stop in improvement on their weight-loss program—they have hit a plateau. My patients often tell me with very frustrated looks on their faces and exasperated tones of voice: "Doc, I am religiously doing all you have told me to do. I've been doing all my exercises, watching what and when I eat, and avoiding lifestyle extremes. So why am I not losing fat or weight? I am doing everything by the book. Help!"

This common problem is caused by hormonal imbalances brought on by your body's internal defenses, which are trying to protect the last few pounds of excess fat. As discussed in Chapter 1, your body is designed to hold on to some extra fat, causing everyone at some time or another to hit some kind of weight-loss plateau, no matter how good his or her diet, exercise, or overall lifestyle plan has been. (For more on identifying and overcoming weight-loss plateaus, see Chapter 5.)

The good news is that there are some natural, over-the-counter supplements that are effective at boosting your fat-burning hormones. Some unmistakable signs that hormonal imbalances are responsible for your plateau are:

- Excessive daytime fatigue or sleepiness
- Poor-quality or fragmented sleep, difficulty falling asleep
- Extreme eating habits: very low appetite or out-of-control hunger and binge eating
- Depressed sex drive or sexual function
- Depression
- Large and continued weight gain after pregnancy with difficulty shedding the excess pounds postpregnancy

If you have reached a tough weight-loss plateau and suffer from one or more of the above symptoms, a hormone-boosting supplement may be an excellent addition to your program.

Creatine

Creatine is a nutrient produced in your body and stored in your muscles as a "muscle food" that provides quick energy reserves for your muscles and helps your body maintain high levels of fat-burning hormones while lifting weights or doing other intense exercise. A combination of creatine and exercise helps you quickly build muscle and burn fat. Creatine is the only supplement in this chapter that is derived from the food you eat. It is naturally found in meat, and your body can produce it using proteins that you eat. But many studies have shown numerous benefits of giving your body extra creatine through supplementation.

Until recently, creatine has been used mainly by male athletes who are trying to build muscle, but it also is an excellent supplement for women trying to lose fat while preserving or building muscle. It is not a "steroid," as the media sometimes make it out to be, and will not cause masculinizing effects or make women overly muscular. Rather, it will help women improve muscle energy levels so that their workouts are better quality and higher intensity.

Creatine also promotes water retention within cells, causing water storage in muscles, which is valuable to dieters who want to build muscle without bloating. Older people also benefit from this effect as it replenishes depleted water within aging cells. With extra hydration, old cells can function more youthfully in terms of their energy production and fat burning. Some people may experience loose stools, but this can be corrected by lowering the dosage. However, this effect is beneficial to relieve constipation.

You should buy creatine in the monohydrate form as opposed to citrate or phosphate, because these forms are often more expensive and their effects not as widely researched. Insulin and carbohydrates help your body absorb creatine, so the best time to take it is with your Magic Window Meal. I recommend a dose of 3 to 5 grams of powder mixed with a small amount of juice every day. Other options are the various high-protein meal replacement drinks and bars that have creatine in them. Take creatine only for two months and then take a month off before beginning the two-month cycle again. While there have been no reports of long-term side effects, many supplements work best when you take them in cycles rather than continuously.

Most people notice improvements in their energy and endurance during workouts after two weeks of supplementation, and improvements in their body after one month. Creatine has been researched extensively and has been shown in repeated studies over the last fifteen years to be safe and highly effective. Because creatine creates significant increases in strength, exercisers need to be careful not to overexert themselves, particularly when lifting weights. Remember to use proper movement and form while lifting weights and to stay within your usual weight parameters.

Some supplement companies recommend that you first start with a one-week "loading" phase of creatine during which you take 10 to 20 grams of creatine in divided doses for seven days, then 3 to 5 grams a day after that. This loading does help if you want to notice the results immediately, but it is not necessary. Your muscles will be fully loaded with creatine if you take 3 to 5 grams a day for three weeks without loading the higher doses, with the same overall effects.

Phosphatidyl Serine

Phosphatidyl serine (PS) is a lipid produced in your brain and is widely available as a natural supplement derived from soybeans. The supplement was first introduced as a brain nutrient to help boost memory and cognitive abilities and is sold as a prescription drug in Europe for treating people with memory disorders. In addition to its positive effects on the nervous system, PS also helps promote an optimal fat-burning hormone environment for those who exercise regularly.

PS is a hormone balancer or regulator that keeps your hormones on a fat-burning track and a muscle-building mode during or after exercise. Over time, aerobic exercise tends to lower the levels of your fat-burning hormones, and people who have been weight training correctly for several months may at some point also experience a drop in the effects of their fat-burning hormones.

Just as the timing of your meals and exercise is extremely important, so is the timing of your PS supplement. When preparing for an aerobic workout, take PS approximately 20 to 30 minutes before you start exercising. You want PS to reach its peak effect around the middle of your workout to keep your body in fat-burning mode. On the days you are weight training, take PS immediately before you lift. Then the peak effect of PS occurs close to the end of your workout and maintains the high levels of fat-burning hormones generated while lifting weights well after your workout is over. PS also corrects the body's tendency (especially in older people) to burn muscle and promote fat storage after lifting weights.

If you have difficulty sleeping, you can take PS at night, about two to three hours before going to bed. Some people who exercise in the evening experience excessive levels of stress hormones before going to bed, resulting in sleeplessness and excessive late-night eating. PS may be effective in promoting rest and relaxation and inducing sleep.

PS has an excellent record not only of effectiveness but also of safety—side effects or complications are extremely rare. Sometimes mild stomach distress occurs from taking large amounts, but this can be avoided by starting with a low dose and gradually increasing it.

The dose for boosting memory and cognitive function is quite affordable at 100 to 200 milligrams per day. But the hormone-balancing dose is much higher at about 400 milligrams a day for women and 600 milligrams for men, although you will have to experiment to find the most effective dosage, especially if you are overweight. Do not exceed 800 milligrams per day without medical supervision.

PS is very expensive, but you can save money by taking your full dose only on days that you exercise or on days you feel out of control from stress. For nonexercising days, take either a maintenance dose of 100 to 200 milligrams, or none at all. Also, take PS in a cyclical on-off fashion, just as you would take creatine. In general, most performance-enhancing supplements work best if you give your body a break from them from time to time and only use them for four to eight weeks at a time.

Androdiol

Androdiol is the brand name of the prohormone 4-androstenediol (4AD). Prohormones are naturally occurring compounds in the body and are sold over the counter in supplement form. Prohormones are highly effective at promoting temporary boosts of fat-burning hormones such as testosterone. Unlike PS, which works through the nervous system to balance and regulate your hormones, prohormones work by providing your body with raw materials to produce more of its own natural hormones. Prohormones are perhaps the most powerful and effective supplements currently available for promoting increased energy, better workouts, improved mood, and increased sex drive. Most important for the Hormone Revolution program, prohormones boost levels of hormones that will help you burn fat and build muscle.

Androdiol is a direct precursor to testosterone. This means that your body converts Androdiol to testosterone in one quick and simple reaction, making it the most effective yet gentlest-acting prohormone supplement. After you take it, you will experience a temporary boost in testosterone levels that will last for three to four hours and help your body stay in fat-burning mode. Higher levels of testosterone can energize your workout, increase your strength and endurance, and help your muscles repair and grow.

Androdiol is quite safe if used appropriately and not abused. It produces only a temporary spike in hormone levels and does not disturb your body's natural hormone production or run the risk of signaling the brain to reduce its natural sex hormone production. When abused, synthetic injectable anabolic steroids can cause the body's natural testosterone production to shut down almost completely for prolonged periods of time. HDL cholesterol (good cholesterol) levels can go down severely as well. Both of these effects are less of a risk when using natural potent prohormones such as Androdiol. However, even when using natural testosterone-boosting supplements, I still recommend being cautious and following the guidelines below.

Men should take 100 to 200 milligrams of Androdiol 20 to 30 minutes before working out, three to four times per week. Those who are using a sublingual (under the tongue) Androdiol lozenge can decrease their dosage to 12 to 25 milligrams. Androdiol users should cycle their doses, taking it for four to six weeks, then abstaining for the same amount of time they were on it. Men who are older (more than thirty to forty years old) should use Androdiol for even shorter periods and take more time off to get the best results.

Some bodybuilders and athletes take multiple doses of Androdiol every day of the week. While these larger doses can be effective for building muscle and burning fat, this approach is only recommend for experienced and/or younger weight lifters with at least one to two years of dedicated training. People who have just started working out need only a little boost and do not have to bombard their bodies with a constant barrage of extra hormones. If you do decide to take larger doses, seek medical supervision and have regular blood tests for hormone levels, cholesterol levels, and liver function. While there have been few reported side effects from people using Androdiol, whenever using large doses of a supplement or a drug that impacts hormone levels, you should be on the lookout for potential prostate problems, acne, and lowered HDL cholesterol levels.

Androdiol is a mild hormone booster for men but is very potent when used by women. Far fewer women than men take Androdiol because it is rarely sold in doses appropriate for them to take. Whereas men may need up to 200 milligrams of Androdiol, women should only take 5 to 25 milligrams two to three times a week, or 1 to 5 milligrams if taken as a sublingual lozenge. Women should start out with a very small dose of about 5 milligrams and increase it slowly by 5 milligrams at a time, up to a maximum dosage of 25 milligrams per day. There are a few products available in powder or a liquid spray that grant greater flexibility with dosages. Some women also use a pill cutter to cut a 12-milligram lozenge in three or four pieces of about 3 to 4 milligrams each. Women should take Androdiol in cycles of two to four weeks.

Young women still wishing to have children should not take Androdiol or any other prohormone. As with birth control pills, usage of prohormones can make conceiving later in life much more difficult. Women who experience acne (which is rare at the doses I recommend) should reduce their dose immediately. Another alternative is to use DHEA (discussed later in this chapter), which is a much milder prohormone.

Hormone Boosters and Aging

Hormone-boosting supplements should enhance your diet and exercise program and help you overcome weight-loss plateaus, but they are not enough to correct long-term hormonal imbalances that result from aging. For some people, taking PS or Androdiol results in excessively strong hormone boosts that greatly decrease fatigue or soreness after exercise, promotes sudden progress in weight loss or muscle building, or triggers rapid weight-training gains in either the amount of weight lifted or the number of repetitions completed. Making slow, steady advancements is normal, but sudden acceleration in strength and ability after taking a PS or Androdiol is a sign that these supplements are correcting a hormonal imbalance in your body that may be more serious or entrenched than you think. If you are in your forties or older and seem to be getting disproportionate results from hormone-boosting supplements, you may want to have your doctor check your sex hormone levels. In the next chapter we will discuss proven methods of fighting age-related hormonal imbalances and how overcoming them can be an effective way to break through your weight-loss plateaus.

THERMOGENICS

Thermogenics are natural supplements that stimulate your nervous system and can give you more energy for exercising. They actually increase fat burning within your body by raising your body's temperature. The most common thermogenic supplements are the herbs ma huang (ephedrine) and guarana (caffeine), green tea, and forskolin. Unlike the supplements in the Core Supplement program, thermogenics should only be taken for a specified amount of time as plateau breakers.

A description of the thermogenic agents is given below, along with instructions on how to take them individually and in conjunction with one another. It is particularly important that you review not only the benefits of thermogenics but also the precautions, as supplements containing ephedrine are not for everyone and should be taken with a great deal of caution.

Benefits

Most weight-loss drugs or supplements work though only one mechanism, but thermogenics help you burn fat, lose weight, and break through weight-loss plateaus in four important ways: They increase your metabolism, preserve muscle, decrease your appetite, and increase your energy. Keep in mind that you still have to stay on the Hormone Revolution Weight-Loss Plan and exercise program while taking thermogenics; the thermogenic metabolism boost alone cannot make up for poor eating and lifestyle choices.

Your body's metabolism naturally tends to slow down while you are restricting calories. As mentioned before, thermogenics boost your body's temperature, leading to a faster metabolism with more fat being burned. Studies have shown that thermogenics are highly effective not only at increasing your metabolism but also at focusing it on burning fat rather than muscle. One study showed that dieters not on thermogenics who lost weight lost roughly half from burning muscle, but those taking thermogenics lost almost 90 percent of the weight they lost from burning fat. This means you can burn off around twice the amount of fat while preserving muscle. People on thermogenics also experience a large reduction in appetite and are far less likely to overeat. Thermogenics are perhaps the most potent energizing supplements available over the counter, and people who take them tend to be more active overall throughout the day. Taking thermogenics prior to exercise can enhance your workout intensity and its duration.

Precautions

The FDA has been trying unsuccessfully for a long time to ban or restrict ephedrine-containing supplements because of many of these precautions. But it has failed mostly because it has not had adequate scientific evidence to support its actions. In fact, Congress severely reprimanded the FDA for issuing a negative report on ephedrine that was full of factual errors. The FDA's campaign against ephedrine has been based on politics, not science, as evidenced by its long history of attacking supplements that threaten the prescription pharmaceutical industry. Further safety reviews have been ordered by the government, and I expect them to confirm my conclusion that ephedrine actually has much stronger safety and efficacy records that any prescription weight-loss drug such as Meridia or Orlistat. I also believe the review will find that ephedrine is safe and effective for weight loss if the right precautions are taken and if it is taken under the supervision of your physician.

Thermogenics have many benefits for a lot of people, but they are not for everyone. While thermogenics have a generally good safety record, they are not to be taken by people who are in poor health, pregnant, under eighteen, or are frail or elderly. People with high blood pressure, seizure or neurological disorders, chest pain, heart or thyroid problems, diabetes, nervousness, poor sleep, or psychiatric disorders should not take thermogenics or supplements containing ephedrine. Although thermogenics are over-the-counter natural supplements, they should be treated like drugs. Always read the label of any thermogenic supplement carefully. Discontinue use and consult a physician in the event of dizziness or other contraindications. And most important, make sure your doctor knows that you are taking these supplements.

Thermogenics already have a strong dose of caffeine, so you should greatly limit or avoid beverages or other products containing caffeine. The main side effects of thermogenics, like caffeine, are nervousness and jitters. Some people can minimize this by starting with a low dose, but others simply cannot tolerate the effects of thermogenics. If you cannot drink a cup of high-quality coffee (200 to 250 milligrams of caffeine) without jittery or nervous side effects, then you should not use thermogenics. These products are not compatible with your system.

Ma Huang

Ma huang is a natural source of the powerful thermogenic agent ephedrine and has been used in Chinese medicine for thousands of years. Ephedrine is perhaps the single most potent naturally occurring thermogenic agent, and therefore it is important to strictly regulate your dosage. Because of its potency, make sure you buy ma huang from a reputable supplement company that contains a high-quality, standardized ma huang extract to ensure precise dosage and maximization of the effects.

There are less-stimulating thermogenic formulas available that usually replace ma huang with synephrine, a less potent stimulant that comes from bitter oranges. There are far fewer studies on synephrine than on ma huang and ephedrine. Synephrine usually does not make people jittery the same way ma huang does, but it is not nearly as effective. Those who can't handle ma huang should take a simple green tea extract supplement instead.

Be sure to closely read the labels of any thermogenic product you buy. Most reliable brands sell thermogenics with 330 milligrams of ma huang extract standardized for 6 percent ephedrine alkaloids (ephedrine and related compounds), which gives you 20 milligrams of ephedrine alkaloids per serving. The FDA recommends only 8 milligrams of ephedrine per dose and only 24 milligrams total per day. Health Canada, the Canadian equivalent of the FDA, recommends dosage limits to 8 milligrams per dose, for a maximum dosage of 32 milligrams per day for no more than seven days, and has issued a voluntary recall on all supplements that were not labeled accordingly. While many scientific studies have shown that healthy people can take larger doses safely, the FDA and Health Canada guidelines are a good place to start, and you can discuss dosage increases with your doctor. Before you begin to take ma huang, or any thermogenic, visit your doctor to check for blood pressure or heart problems.

Guarana

Guarana, a berry grown in South America, is a good source of the most common thermogenic agent, caffeine. Some thermogeric formulas use kola nut as an alternative source of caffeine. By itself, caffeine is a relatively mild thermogenic—you might notice a small increase in your body temperature after drinking coffee or a caffeinated soft drink. But combined in a thermogenic formula with ma huang, guarana has a more potent effect than caffeine or ma huang when taken alone (discussed above). Most good thermogenic products are standardized to have roughly 200 milligrams of caffeine per serving. I recommend a maximum of 400 milligrams of guarana a day, taken in two doses at least four hours apart. If you are caffeine sensitive, you should avoid taking guarana before bedtime or possibly at all.

Green Tea

While ma huang and guarana are the main ingredients in most thermogenics supplements, there are usually additional ingredients found in most formulas. One of the most healthful thermogenic ingredients is green tea extract. Studies have shown that green tea and its extract have strong anti-cancer properties and can improve cardiovascular health. But the main reason green tea extract is included in thermogenic formulas is that it has fat-burning effects.

Green tea extract has strong effects on your metabolism, partially because of its small caffeine content, which leads to more fat burning and muscle preservation. But most of this effect is due to the unique actions of compounds in green tea called *polyphenols,* which help your body mobilize fatty acids to use as energy rather than muscle. Try to find a thermogenic product with green tea extract standardized for at least 200 milligrams of polyphenols per serving. Given the many diverse health benefits of a complete thermogenic formula, those who choose not to use one should take green tea extract by itself.

Forskolin

Forskolin *(Coleus forskohli)* has been used for thousands of years in traditional Indian Ayurvedic medicine. Forskolin is included as a fat burner in most thermogenic formulas because it has been shown to be effective in boosting thyroid hormones and may help elevate testosterone levels. It also has a calming, relaxing effect, which lowers your blood pressure and helps balance out the highly stimulating effects of ma huang and caffeine (both of which can raise your blood pressure). Multithermogenic formulas typically contain an extract standardized for 5 to 10 milligrams of forskolin per serving.

One small warning: Forskolin can have prosexual effects, such as promoting erections. My male patients and their partners usually consider this a positive side effect!

How to Use Thermogenics

The first rule for thermogenic use is to get your diet, lifestyle, and exercise habits in order before taking them. I only recommend thermogenics to people who have already been following the Hormone Revolution program carefully and who have been making steady progress for at least three to six months. It is only after you have hit a plateau following initial progress that thermogenics should be used. Otherwise, you are not the correct candidate or at the right point in your weight-loss plan to qualify for thermogenic use.

If you have not made weight-loss progress and have not become healthy or fit, then thermogenics could have a greater likelihood of adverse effects. Review the precautions above and speak to your physician to determine if you should take thermogenics.

In addition to its use as part of a thermogenic formula, forskolin can be taken individually to boost a weight-loss program or to lower blood pressure. The maximum dose of forskolin I recommend is 20 milligrams per day (from 200 milligrams of *Coleus forskohli*). Of course, as with any supplement, you should discuss your usage with a knowledgeable physician or health care practitioner before taking it.

Choose a thermogenic product from a reputable company (such as those recommended in Appendix II) so that you can be sure it meets the claims on the label. Some supplement companies try to cut costs by using lower-quality ma huang and guarana extracts, in which case you will not know if the product has too much or too little caffeine and ephedrine. The main ingredients in a thermogenic formula are ma huang and ephedrine; more effective and healthful higher-end thermogenic formulas will also contain forskolin and green tea extract.

Thermogenics should not be taken every day but in a cyclical fashion. You can experience the benefits of thermogenics even if you take them only two days a week. I recommend taking them for four to five days a week, and then going off for at least two days per week. After taking thermogenics for two months, you should then discontinue use for a month. The appetite-suppressing effects of thermogenics diminish if you take them for too long without taking a break. You also should not become dependent on thermogenics for losing weight—they should be used only to get you past a plateau in your workout, after which you should discontinue their use. Taking thermogenics in a cyclical fashion will help you get the maximum effect from thermogenics with the minimum amount of stress on your body.

When beginning to take thermogenic supplements, whether individually or in combination, start with a low dose and gradually build it up. If you choose to take a supplement that combines multiple thermogenics in one product, find one that divides the dosages into at least three capsules per dose. This way, you will be able to start with one-third of the dose suggested on the bottle and slowly work your way up to a full dose. Some products recommend taking three doses per day, but I find that can be excessive and suggest taking them only twice daily—once in the morning and once at noon or in the midafternoon. If you exercise in the morning, it is best to use them one hour prior to exercise once a day and then again before three in the afternoon.

Bottom Line

When used correctly by healthy people, thermogenics can be like rocket fuel for the final few pounds of fat that you are trying to lose. They are especially useful for people whose progress is impeded by fatigue or hunger. If you are already following the diet and exercise plans in this book, taking these supplements should give you a huge boost. You should notice increased energy, better sleep, and less muscle soreness. Also, you should notice that you are making better and faster progress over time—less fat, more muscle.

FIVE

MONITORING YOUR SUCCESS

Finding ways to monitor your progress is an extremely important aspect of sticking with your program. We look at ourselves in the mirror every day and often don't notice the small decreases in weight and fat that are slowly occurring, causing many people to think they are not making progress or to fail to notice that they are not achieving what they should. Knowing exactly how much progress, or how little, you are making is the best way to stay motivated in your diet and exercise program.

WEIGHT-LOSS PLATEAUS

No matter how consistent your diet, exercise, and supplement program is, your body will build up a tremendous defense against hormone stimulation and a fortified resistance against further weight and fat loss—a plateau. The trick to overcoming this is to identify as soon as possible whether you have actually reached a true hormonal plateau or if you have simply strayed from your Hormone Revolution Weight-Loss Plan.

A true or authentic weight-loss plateau occurs when you experience weight loss and fitness stop or slowdowns after three to six months of noticeable progress even though you have not changed anything in your program. You cannot say you have reached a true plateau unless you have first made some solid, long-term progress. If you have reached a plateau, first pat yourself on the back for making solid progress for several months. Then you should consider implementing some of the plateau-breaking hormone-booster supplements described in Chapter 4 or adjusting your exercise program through periodization or other methods as outlined in Chapter 2.

However, if you experience few or no results in the program, then you need to take a good look at how you have structured your exercise and diet plans. Monitoring your Hormone Revolution Weight-Loss Plan is the best way to achieve results, by ensuring that you stick to it at all times. Below are several methods for monitoring the success of your program, and some troubleshooting tips.

MONITORING YOUR EXERCISE PROGRESS

Exercise Log

An exercise log is a journal that records your compliance with your exercise program. Carry this log with you whenever you go to the gym, and look back on it on days that you don't exercise to look for holes or weaknesses in your training. In this log, you should keep track of:

1. Which exercises you did and the time of day you did them to monitor how closely you are sticking to your program.
2. Number of weight-lifting sets and reps, along with the amount of weight used for each set to track your gains in strength.

3. Calories burned and steps or miles covered during aerobic exercise (you will need a Digiwalker or a Calorie Tracker) to gauge the efficiency of your aerobic exercise.

4. Morning heart rate when still in bed to ensure that you are not overtraining or suffering from hormonal imbalance. If your heart rate is over 80 to 95, you should scale back your training program and talk to your doctor.

5. General notes about how you felt after exercising (e.g., full of energy, out of breath, exhausted, etc.) to guard against unhealthy patterns of fatigue or exhaustion, which indicate overtraining or hormone imbalance.

If you are not making the progress you think you should, look for clues as to why in your log, especially where you record your weight-training performance. Ideally, you should be getting stronger and making slow but steady increases in the amount of weight you lift. If you see that you have been missing workouts, then your problem is undertraining. Exhaustion and fatigue after exercise most likely mean that you are overtraining. Also ask your training buddy or personal trainer to look at your log for a second opinion. Make the necessary adjustments until you are back on track and making progress.

Troubleshooting

When many people begin formally exercising on a set program for the first time, they often get discouraged either by the difficulty of the program or by a lack of results. Several of these problems are due to improper technique or overtraining and can be easily corrected. Following are some tips for diagnosing and solving three common exercise problems:

· **Prolonged muscle soreness:** If your muscles are always sore, even several days after exercising, you are clearly overtraining. Try giving yourself more rest between weight-lifting days and slightly lower the intensity of your exercise by lifting lighter weights. Once you are at a point that pain and soreness go away quickly after lifting weights, you can slowly start increasing the amount of weight you lift each session.

- **No increases in strength:** If you don't have any pain or soreness and seem to be recovering from exercise well but are not seeing any increases in strength, chances are you are eating improperly and are losing muscle. Try eating your Magic Window Meal (discussed in Chapter 3) more quickly after you work out, and make sure you are getting enough protein in your overall diet.
- **Increases in strength, but not in muscle mass:** One common solution to this problem is to drink a low-carbohydrate protein shake with 25 to 35 grams of protein immediately before exercising. Ingesting protein right before lifting weights is an excellent way to directly feed amino acids into your muscles during the weight-training period.

Injuries and the Role of Physical Therapy

Major and minor injuries can easily derail any weight-loss program: Pain can quickly cause you to lose your motivation. But both can be overcome and actually remedied by fitness and exercise. It also is important to take steps to avoid minor injuries that can occur with exercise. At some point in life, most people eventually develop some problem with their joints or spine, especially as they age. Sometimes you can work around these problems if they are minor, but, in order to achieve maximum results from your training and to keep your body healthy, you need to ensure that you are injury free. To do this, you may require the help of a physical therapist. Below is a list of some common indications that you may require physical therapy:

1. You feel a distinct line of shooting pain or numbness down one or both arms or legs. This also can be associated with an odd sensation, numbness, or tingling, indicating that you have a pinched nerve that

deserves medical attention. The most common cause is a herniated disc in the neck or lower back.

2. Localized intense pain in an extremity
3. Loss of full range of motion of a joint
4. Any type of pain that keeps you from sleeping
5. Joints that sublux, or dislocate (go out of their normal socket)
6. Untreated high blood pressure or cardiac disease

If you have any of these problems, they should be treated before starting or continuing the Hormone Revolution Exercise Plan. Oftentimes, you can train with a physical therapist even after your injury is healed. Sometimes you may need to return to your doctor or physical therapist to readjust the program if your problem persists.

MONITORING YOUR DIETARY PROGRESS

Food Log

Most people cheat on their diets far more than they realize. If you are cheating on your diet more than once or twice per week, your progress might be greatly slowed down. Remember, cheating on the Hormone Revolution program not only means that you are eating the wrong foods but also that you are eating the right foods at the wrong times. Keeping a daily food log that includes all your meals and snacks (including beverages) from morning to night is the best way to monitor your diet and guard against cheating.

At the bottom of each page containing your daily meals, write a separate list of any items that were "cheat foods" in your diet. This includes any sugary or starchy foods not eaten during the Magic Window or eaten too much during the Magic Window, such as most snack chips, pastries, candies, fast food, and pretty much any other food high in processed starches, sugars, saturated fats, or trans-fats. During the first week on the Hormone Revolution program, when you have begun exercising but not dieting, cheat foods might account for practically all of your meals. You may be doing a lot of writing during your first week!

During the second and third weeks, you should be listing fewer and fewer foods on your cheat list. If you are exercising regularly, you might be surprised by how your cheat-food consumption drops without much thought—almost like you are eating healthier automatically. By the fourth week, you should have practically no cheat foods listed in your log.

If writing down everything you eat every day seems silly to you, think again. People are much more likely to stick with their diets when they are paying close attention to what they eat. It is when you stop thinking so much about your diet that you are likely to slip. This also will be valuable information when troubleshooting problems in achieving your weight-loss goals. Keeping a diet log is crucial to long-term success on the Hormone Revolution diet.

Weighing In

Of course, the primary indicator of your success on the Hormone Revolution program will be your weight. When beginning on the eating plan, you should use a standard scale to measure your weight every day, at the same time of day. Because your weight can fluctuate throughout the day, you should weigh yourself either first thing in the morning or right before you go to bed. Write down your weight in your eating log so you can follow your long-term trends.

After you have lost an initial 5 to 10 pounds, or when you begin the second month of the program, you should start using a body-fat scale (for more information, see the section "Body-Fat Scales" later in this chapter), which measures the percentage of your weight that is from fat, instead of a standard weight scale. This method will be more accurate in recording your progress as it can help you ensure that you are losing weight due to fat loss, not muscle loss (see the "Troubleshooting" section below if you suspect your weight loss is not due to a decrease in your body fat). Again, it is important to measure your body fat at the same time of day every day in order to get consistent measurements. Each day you should record your body-fat measurement in your log.

When recording your first measurements with a body-fat scale, you should also make some additional calculations. You will need a calculator to measure two key indicators of your progress: (1) your total body fat in pounds, and (2) your lean (nonfat) body weight in pounds. You can calculate your total body fat simply by multiplying your body-fat percentage by your total weight. For example, if you weigh 160 pounds and your body-fat percentage is 25 percent, then your total body-fat weight would be:

$$.25 \times 160 = 40 \text{ pounds}$$

Your lean body weight is simply your total weight minus your body-fat weight. In this example, your lean body weight would be:

$$160 - 40 = 120 \text{ pounds}$$

Good progress is marked by decreasing body-fat weight and a constant or decreasing lean body weight. This means that you are losing fat while gaining or preserving muscle mass. An ideal body-fat percentage for men is 10 to 15 percent and 15 to 20 percent for women. An ideal goal to achieve this result is to try to lose ½ to 1 pound of body-fat weight per week.

If you do not want to buy a body-fat measurement scale, you can have your body fat measured using the skin-caliper method, which can be performed by an experienced personal trainer or health professional. While the skin-caliper method is not especially accurate, it can be useful for detecting long-term trends if a knowledgeable person makes the measurements on a regular basis.

Troubleshooting

So what should you do if you are not making the progress you think you should be making on your Hormone Revolution Eating Plan? Below is a list of common pitfalls and my diagnosis and prescription for overcoming them.

Your Body-Fat and Lean Body Weight Are Going Down: This could indicate that you are losing both muscle and fat. The most likely cause of this is that you are not eating enough protein. Make sure you eat at least 30 grams of protein during your Magic Window Meal, and at least 1 gram of protein per pound of your lean body weight in four to six divided portions per day. You also might want to try drinking a high-protein/low-carbohydrate shake before your workouts.

You Are Not Losing Any Body-Fat Weight: If you fail to lose any body-fat weight for two weeks in a row in spite of the regular exercise and dieting recommended in Chapter 2, you should take a careful look at your diet logs: There may be hidden sources of calories in your food. Here are some solutions to some of the most common calorie impediments to success:

- The most common sources of hidden calories are sauces and cooking oils. Make sure you are using only the low-calorie sauces suggested in Chapter 3. Also, make sure you are not eating too many fried foods or eating too many of your meals (more than two a week) at restaurants.
- Strictly limit all starch and moderate- and low-fiber foods (even some fruits and vegetables) to the postworkout Magic Window Meal only. Also keep your consumption of oil, even canola oil and olive oil, to an absolute minimum. Once you start losing weight again, you can begin to slowly add servings of fruits and moderate-fiber vegetables, along with small amounts of healthy oils, back to your diet. This further adjustment of your diet is just a temporary "emergency" measure to get your progress back on track.

- If all else fails, count calories. I am not a huge fan of calorie counting, but for some people it is the only way to flush out hidden calorie sources. If you are preparing your own meals, estimating your daily calorie intake should be quite easy. There are numerous books and websites (see the web resources in the back of this book) that give calorie counts of common foods. Also designer foods such as high-protein bars and meal-replacement drinks have accurate calorie counts on the labels. Likely, you will find that your excess calories do not come from vegetables or lean sources of protein, but from other sources. If you are a man of average weight (170 to 175 pounds), make sure your calorie count is around 2,000 per day or less. If you are a woman of average weight (110 to 130 pounds), make sure your calorie count is around 1,600 per day. To calculate the minimum amount of calories you should be eating, multiply your lean body weight by thirteen.

Extreme Hunger and Insomnia at Night: Many people on diets find themselves starving and unable to sleep. Bedtime is when we are often most vulnerable to cheating on our diets. I have designed my program the best way possible to avoid this problem, but if you are finding it difficult to sleep at night here are some suggestions:

- Eat before you go to sleep! You probably have been told that eating before you go to bed is fattening, but this is only true if you overeat or eat the wrong foods (starch or carbohydrates). Eating some protein, like a protein bar or a small bowl of nonfat cottage cheese, before bed can help stop your nighttime hunger and provide your body with fuel to repair and build muscle while you sleep.
- If you are highly anxious at night, then you can make the exception of occasionally eating one piece of toast or two to three crackers with your late-night protein meal. This may calm you down for better sleep.

- Try taking the supplement 5 hydroxy-tryptophan (5HTP) to calm down and get better sleep. This supplement also can help some people with carbohydrate cravings.
- Eat a larger breakfast. People who eat a small breakfast or skip it entirely are most likely to have hunger cravings later in the day.

THE LATEST TECHNOLOGY

Modern technology has created many new inventions that can be useful for tracking your progress on the Hormone Revolution program. Body-fat scales, calorie-tracking machines, and the Internet can help you measure more accurately how your program is working and determine what you need to do to make better progress.

Body-Fat Scales

Most people track their progress while on a diet and exercise program the old-fashioned way—by using their regular weighing scale. While this is efficient for the first four weeks of the program, a regular weight scale will become an increasingly inaccurate measure of your progress as your diet progresses. During the first month of the diet program, body-fat scale measurements will actually be imprecise because they are highly dependent on a consistent amount of water in your body. Both exercise and protein consumption cause your body to lose water, and most of your initial weight loss will come from this water loss as your body adjusts to the new program. But once your body becomes accustomed to your weight-loss program and you begin making progress, regular scales can actually obscure the results of your diet and exercise.

Your weight can fluctuate as much as 5 to 10 pounds throughout the week and even throughout the day, depending on what and how much you eat and drink and the kind of exercise you do, among other things. For obese people, this number can be even higher. Most of these fluctuations are due to changes in water weight and have nothing to do with calories or fat loss. Although after the first month of the program you will have a more standard amount of water in your body, additional fluctuations throughout the week will make standard weight measurements useless, thus necessitating an alternative method for measuring fat and muscle in your body.

As mentioned before, an inappropriate diet and exercise program can lead to loss of muscle and can actually make you fatter. While losing weight in this way might make you feel good in the short term, you could actually be increasing the amount of fat in your body without knowing it. Weighing yourself on a standard scale will not tell you if you are losing pounds as a result of fat loss or muscle loss, which could jeopardize your fitness.

You also can make tremendous progress on the program without losing any weight at all. Because muscle weighs more than fat, you could be building valuable fat-burning muscle and losing fat while not losing actual pounds. While your fitness is improving, by weighing yourself on a scale you could be fooled into becoming disillusioned with your program.

The solution to these problems is to measure your body-fat percentage—the total amount of fat in your body as a percentage of your total body weight—instead of your weight. You can decrease your body-fat percentage either by losing fat without losing muscle or by gaining muscle while retaining fat. As previously mentioned, healthy ranges of body-fat percentages are about 15 to 20 percent for women and 10 to 15 percent for men.

Until recently, measuring body-fat percentage was quite difficult and expensive. People often had to rely on crude techniques such as the skin-caliper test that estimates body fat based on the thickness of your skin, or the "dunk tank" method that measures body fat based on your underwater body weight. These measurements are difficult, expensive, and full of errors and require a great deal of expertise and accuracy.

Recent technology has made available many options for easy, accurate, and inexpensive methods of measuring your body-fat percentage. The most accurate method for measuring body fat utilizes the dual-energy X-ray absorptiometry (DEXA) scanning machine. After it scans your entire body, the DEXA gives you a comprehensive printout that shows your total body-fat percentage and the distribution of your body fat in each part of your body while also measuring your bone density. DEXA measurements can help ensure that you are losing body fat while maintaining or increasing bone density and muscle mass while on my program. The DEXA is extremely accurate, but unfortunately it costs about $200 per measurement, and there is some minimal X-ray exposure involved, making weekly use unrealistic. However, those who are at risk for or who have developed osteoporosis would particularly benefit from this measurement once or twice a year, and it may be covered by insurance.

Fortunately, there are less expensive and more convenient devices to measure your body-fat percentage. One company has developed weighing scales that measure your body-fat percentage through bioelectrical impedance analysis (BIA). These scales cost between $70 and $200, depending on the model, and are very easy to use. After entering your age, weight, gender, and height, you step barefoot on the machine and it measures your weight and the amount of water in your body. In a matter of seconds, the BIA scale will generate an estimate of your body-fat percentage.

While BIA is not nearly as accurate as the DEXA technology, it is consistent in its measurements. Even if the scale overestimates or underestimates your body-fat percentage, it is consistent enough to accurately tell you if your body-fat percentage is increasing or decreasing. By tracking the trends in the measurements it generates, you will be able to get an accurate reading of the amount of body fat you gain or lose based on the initial reading from the machine. For example, suppose in reality your body-fat percentage is 15 percent, but the machine tells you it is 17 percent. If your body fat drops a percentage point, the machine will then tell you that it is 16 percent. While this number is inaccurate, the machine is correct in indicating your progress, in that your body-fat percentage has dropped by 1 percentage point. BIA body-fat scales will enable you to track your progress while on the Hormone

Revolution Weight-Loss Plan, which is the most important measurement you'll need.

Getting a consistent reading of your body-fat percentage relies heavily on obtaining your measurements at the same time of day. The manufacturers suggest that you only take your measurement in the evening with an empty bladder before going to bed. While the exact time of day is probably not important, it is imperative to take your measurement at roughly the same time of day every day to get a consistent measurement.

Calorie-Tracking Machines

Measuring the precise number of calories you are burning while you exercise and also during the nonexercising portions of the day can be invaluable for tracking your progress on the Hormone Revolution program. In the past, we have had to estimate how many calories we burn, based on the types of exercise we perform and how long we do them. Some aerobic exercising machines, such as treadmills and stair climbers, give you an estimate of the number of calories burned based on your weight, the intensity of your exercise, and the amount of time you exercise. However, these are all just rough estimates and can be highly inaccurate. In addition, the effectiveness of these exercises varies greatly from person to person.

There are now small calorie-tracking devices that you can wear while you exercise that can give you highly accurate measurements of the amount of calories you are burning during your workout. These devices are usually worn at the hip area and make accurate assessments of the calories you burn based on your leg movements. This device also can be used to estimate the number of calories burned, steps taken, and the distance walked while doing everyday tasks such as walking to the corner store, mowing the lawn, or raking the leaves.

If you are not losing as much weight or fat as you think you should relative to how much you exercise, you should consider buying one of these devices. Effective aerobic exercise should burn 7 to 10 calories per minute. Any more than this and you might be overtraining and causing too much loss of muscle; any less and you might not be exercising intensely enough. A calorie-tracking device can help you fine-tune your exercise routine to find the right exercises at the right intensity. It also can help you determine how physically active you are during the nonexercising periods of your day.

The Internet

The Internet can be an extremely useful tool for accessing additional health and fitness information and also for enhancing the usefulness of the equipment you use for exercising. While it is not wise to rely on medical information disseminated from the Internet because of the unreliability of its sources and the lack of personal, individual assessment, it is possible to find useful supplemental information for your diet, in particular, as well as for some aspects of your exercise program on the Internet.

One of the calorie-tracking devices even allows you to plug the device into your computer and go to a special webpage where you can download data from the device and produce charts and graphs to illustrate your daily and weekly progress. You can do research on gyms and personal trainers in your area on the Internet.

I personally do not give medical advice over the Internet, as it is impossible to measure heart rate or temperature or to take any other physical measurement online. While giving medical advice online is generally looked down upon by the medical community, online dieting advice has become more and more acceptable. Many good dietitians and nutritionists can provide you with solid dieting advice over the Internet. It is often difficult to find times to meet with a dietitian or nutritionist, and getting advice over the Internet or by e-mail allows you a much more flexible schedule. It is a good idea to meet face-to-face at least once, and then you can maintain regular contact through e-mail or the telephone. Many websites also have wonderful recipe ideas, and you can chat and receive support from other dieters.

There are some precautions you should be aware of regarding Internet dieting. Be discriminating when choosing which site to use (see the web resources in the back of this book for information on specific websites). Avoid sites that try to sell you products, as the validity of their nutritional advice is prejudiced by their motivation to make a sale. Also, some people remain inactive for far too long during the day because of surfing on the Internet. Those who already turn to the Internet as a result of boredom, loneliness, and depression are also those most likely to overeat. Finding exercise buddies and friends with whom to exchange recipes and diet tips will enhance your program far more than relying entirely on the Internet.

SIX

LIFESTYLE AND AGING

The Hormone Revolution program is a complete lifestyle program. This chapter will discuss how many choices in your daily life influence the hormones that contribute to fat burning and aging. Stress and medications can influence the effectiveness of your fat-burning hormones. In this chapter you will learn how to adapt your living habits in order to harness the power of your hormones for optimal weight loss and take advantage of the many additional benefits you will learn about in the next chapter.

This chapter also will discuss the impact of aging on your hormones, particularly the periods in life known as menopause and andropause (male menopause). Men and women alike experience a drop in levels of their fat-burning hormones during midlife. While these events often have many negative connotations, among them weight gain, the drop in hormone production is a natural occurrence that can actually have health benefits. Careful planning through the Hormone Revolution program at this point in your midlife can help you advance your weight-loss and fitness program.

STRESS

Leading a stimulating lifestyle that allows you to set new goals and meet new challenges is healthy for your body. Striving to excel in the workplace, sports, relationships, or any area of life is a generally positive way to lead your life emotionally and physically. As you participate in challenging and even competitive activities, your testosterone and other hormone levels will rise to help stimulate your body. The fat-burning effects of this surge in hormones is a beneficial by-product of these vigorous lifestyle choices.

Unfortunately, far too many people overextend themselves by working extremely long hours, making too many commitments with their time, and failing to rest, relax, or take vacations. The time demands of these activities can cause a break with social activity, frustration, psychological pressure, obesity, and ill health. Not only are these side effects a result of a stressful lifestyle, they also perpetuate stress, trapping you in unhealthy hormonal patterns.

When you are under stress, your body responds by releasing the hormone cortisol, which actually burns off muscle and promotes fat storage. This effect is exacerbated by the fact that your body decreases its production of testosterone during stressful times. It is important to relieve both the psychological stresses in your life, such as overwork, and the physical stresses on your body, such as alcohol and tobacco, in order to keep your hormones at levels that benefit your fitness and health.

Make sure you make time in your busy schedule to relax. No matter how important the stressful activities in your life are, you are only subverting your efforts and your health by overexerting yourself. You will perform better in the workplace or in any area of life in long run if you make time to clear your head and relax. Taking time to enjoy yourself by socializing with friends, relaxing with your loved ones, taking vacations, or having sex are all essential for minimizing stress. Even some forms of exercise such as yoga (non-Pilates) also can be a very effective way to relax and clear your head.

However, you also must be careful to relieve stress only in healthy ways.

You should never attempt to relieve stress by consuming alcohol or smoking cigarettes. In addition to the possibility of dependence and abuse, using these substances imposes physical stresses on your body. Calories from alcohol are easily converted to fat, often resulting in the beer-belly phenomenon. Even worse, alcohol can sabotage your fat-burning hormones by causing more testosterone to be converted to estrogen. One or two drinks per day, preferably of red wine, can reduce the risk of heart disease and help you relax and enjoy your meals. But anyone serious about losing weight and fat should avoid having more than two drinks per day.

One reason many people smoke is because they think it will help them stay thin. While nicotine can induce a small increase in your metabolism, in the long run smoking is counterproductive to losing weight. Studies have shown that smoking can cause your testosterone levels to decrease and your estrogen levels to increase, resulting in an increase of fat storage. Additional disadvantages also range from the obvious risk of lung cancer to sexual dysfunction in men. By eliminating these physical stresses on your body, you will increase your potential for success on the Hormone Revolution Weight-Loss Plan.

MEDICATION

When you are prescribed a prescription medication, your doctor or pharmacist probably makes you aware of any side effects that the drug may have. You and your doctor probably discuss the contraindications appearing on the label or any other medications you may be taking. But one thing you probably don't discuss is an issue often overlooked by physicians and their patients—the effects of the medication on your hormonal systems. Unfortunately, many common prescription drugs can disrupt your fat-burning hormones and thwart your weight-loss plan. For three common culprits—ulcer, antifungal, and anti-inflammatory medications—there are available alternative drugs that don't disturb your hormones.

The popular ulcer medication Tagamet (cimetidine) is well known to suppress testosterone. As you learned throughout this book, testosterone is essential for burning fat and for building and preserving muscle. Men who suffer from ulcers are often over the age of forty-five, when their testosterone levels have already started to drop because of aging. If you have an ulcer and have been prescribed Tagamet, you may want to talk to your doctor about a new generation of ulcer medications, including Prevacid (lansoprazole) and other gastric acid–secretion inhibitors, that do not suppress your testosterone.

Antifungal drugs such as Diflucan (fluconazole) and Nizoral (ketoconazole) also can be extremely disrupting to your hormones. In fact, Nizoral can actually reduce your testosterone levels to nearly zero if taken in high dosages, and it is actually used in scientific experiments specifically as a testosterone-reducing agent. Talk to your doctor about alternative antifungal drugs, such as Lamisil (terbinafine hydrochloride), that do not affect your hormones.

Various anti-inflammatory drugs, such as prednisone, also can negatively affect your hormonal systems, causing increased fat storage and loss of muscle. Fortunately, Celebrex (celecoxib) and Enbrel (etanercept) will not affect your hormones like prednisone.

While some medical conditions may require you to medicate with drugs that subvert your hormone balance, other conditions allow for a variety of choices that will enable you to discuss hormone-friendly options with your doctor.

SLEEP

Your body has complex cycles that cause your hormone levels to fluctuate over a twenty-four-hour period. Healthy men generally wake up in the morning with an erection, mainly because testosterone levels are at their highest after a good night's sleep. Testosterone levels are at their lowest at night, and men as well as women need adequate sleep in order to provoke this important early morning surge in testosterone release.

At least seven to eight hours of sleep a night are required to allow your body enough time to recuperate from the physical activities, exercise, and other stresses throughout the day. An important part of this restorative process is your body's nocturnal release of human growth hormone (hGH). Growth hormones, which are at their highest levels during sleep, help your body burn fat and muscle throughout the night. Sleep is the best way to overcome the physical stress of fatigue throughout the day and is also vital for nurturing your exercise program by fostering muscle growth.

Toxic Estrogens

You are probably aware of numerous environmental health hazards such as polluted air or foods laced with pesticides and preservatives. But you are likely unaware of the artificial hormones in our environment and food that can poison our bodies by suppressing our natural fat-burning hormones. Products we use and foods we eat every day are full of synthetic chemicals, called *xenoestrogens* (*xeno,* meaning "foreign"), which are structurally similar to natural estrogens. Xenoestrogens can be toxic to our hormone systems and can disrupt the functions of both testosterone and estrogen, enhancing fat storage and suppressing fat burning.

Xenoestrogens have already been linked to infertility in men, and studies are under way to see if hormonal poisoning also leads to prostate cancer. In women, xenoestrogens enhance the effects of prescription estrogens, which in turn leads to maximum fat storage and a huge increase in the risk of breast cancer. I expect future research to find that xenoestrogens promote other types of cancers as well.

Because of their omnipresence in our environment, xenoestrogens are extremely difficult to avoid, but many can be eliminated by simply choosing to eat and use natural products. A recent study even suggests that eating organic foods can increase male sperm counts, most likely as a result of consuming fewer xenoestrogens. The only way to actually combat the xenoestrogens you can't evade is to minimize their effects through optimal hormone function on the Hormone Revolution program.

Common Substances Containing Xenoestrogens

Pesticides

Processed foods

Plastic bottles and cups

Standard laundry detergents and other household cleaning products
  (national brands found in most supermarkets)

Bleached paper products (coffee filters, plates, cups)

Synthetic estrogens in birth control pills and HRT treatments
  (especially those derived from horses)

HORMONES AND AGING

Hormone levels are one of the most reliable and important markers of aging. One of the reasons why weight and fat loss become more difficult as we get older is that levels of testosterone and growth hormone decrease as we age and our insulin system function declines. People who exacerbate this effect by following unhealthy lifestyles while aging will trigger the many negative side effects of aging: decreased libido, impaired sexual function, and loss of energy. The additional hormonal disruption of menopause in women and andropause in men exacerbates these symptoms of aging. However, following the Hormone Revolution Weight-Loss Plan can minimize the negative symptoms of aging and indeed even reverse them.

Defeating Menopausal Weight Gain

You have probably noticed that fat and weight loss become extremely difficult for women as they get older. Around the time of menopause, women are put on a hormonal rollercoaster that often leads to rapid weight gain. The diet, exercise, and supplement programs in this book will eliminate and reduce weight gain, but women also need to know more about what happens to their aging hormones in order to better understand menopause and its negative side effects.

Many women are unaware of this, but menopausal weight gain can actually start up to seven years before menopause. While this transitional period in a woman's life is medically known as perimenopause, I often refer to it as "reverse puberty" because, like adolescence, it is a turbulent period during which sex hormone levels fluctuate up and down. By the time a woman reaches menopause, she is left with very low levels of these hormones, especially testosterone, in her body.

To make matters worse, the medical establishment has proven itself to be quite inept in the treatment of menopause. Commonly prescribed hormone replacement therapy (HRT), which brings sex hormone levels back up to or greater than youthful levels, can actually cause more problems than it solves. Every woman approaching menopause should consult with her doctor about treating the symptoms, remembering that for many women HRT isn't the right solution.

I have spent years developing better treatments for menopausal weight gain. Almost every step in my Hormone Revolution program will help ease the transition to menopause and after. But appropriate diet, exercise, and supplements are not always enough to defeat the powerful forces of menopausal weight gain. My natural alternative hormone-balancing program is designed to give women an extra edge in the battle against menopausal weight gain.

Avoiding Toxic Estrogens

Estrogen can in fact have many health benefits when given to the right group of menopausal women. Estrogen replacement therapy is used to treat hot flashes, reduce the risk of heart disease, slow bone loss, and treat other symptoms of menopause. However, as mentioned, improper estrogen replacement therapy can increase the risk of breast cancer and promote obesity in many women.

Many of the negative side effects of HRT are triggered by the most commonly prescribed estrogen, Premarin, which is not a natural human estrogen but estrogen taken from the urine of pregnant mares. To make matters worse, the common form of progesterone (the female sex hormone that triggers monthly periods) given to women is equally problematic. Instead of natural progesterone, women are usually given the synthetic drug Provera, which may actually increase the risk of heart disease. Provera sometimes causes other side effects as well, such as acne or sleeplessness. Natural progesterone, on the other hand, does not produce these side effects and actually has a soothing, calming effect.

Treatments involving estrogen and progesterone regularly result in bloating, weight gain, and even an increased risk of breast cancer and heart disease. These estrogens are such highly potent fat producers that farmers often inject their livestock with them to help fatten them. As a result, postmenopausal women in the United States are at a very high risk of obesity, perhaps more so than any other demographic group.

Natural Estrogen Therapy

Many postmenopausal women do need some sort of estrogen replacement therapy to treat the symptoms of menopause. Natural estrogen replacement therapy involving phytoestrogens can actually relieve hot flashes and lower the risk of heart disease and maybe osteoporosis while minimizing many of the fattening side effects of synthetic estrogens. Phytoestrogens are naturally occurring estrogenlike compounds found in many plants, the most common among them being black cohosh and soy. They have a chemical structure similar to that of human estrogens and a wide variety of positive effects on the human body. Other sources of phytoestrogens you can easily include in your diet or supplement program include red clover, chickpeas, and dong quai.

Black cohosh is remarkably effective in treating hot flashes as well as other symptoms associated with menopause such as nervous tension and depression. The phytoestrogens found in soy (called *isoflavones*) have been found to have many of the same benefits as human estrogen, such as decreasing the risk of heart disease and relieving hot flashes, insomnia, and mood swings. Soy phytoestrogens, unlike human estrogen, may also *reduce* the risk of breast cancer. Most important for the Hormone Revolution program, phytoestrogens do not have the same fattening effects as human estrogen. By relying on natural phytoestrogens rather than the commonly prescribed horse estrogens, women can reap many of the health benefits of estrogens while avoiding the fattening effects.

If soy and black cohosh do not provide adequate treatment for your hot-flash symptoms, low-dosage natural estrogen replacement may be neccessary. However, you should talk with your doctor about taking small doses of natural estrogens that are bioidentical to those found in our bodies instead of synthetic hormones. It is only common sense to give identical human estrogens to a human, and it is also much better for a woman's overall health. These estrogens also are available in the form of transdermal gels or creams that are applied to the skin, which are preferable to pills because they have a much milder fat-storing effect.

Testosterone and Other Androgens

Surprisingly, I have found that more women are in need of testosterone replacement therapy than men. Even before menopause, a woman's production of testosterone drops almost to zero. Unfortunately, most women are only given estrogen to make up for this deficiency. But testosterone and estrogen work best when they are both present in the body in a youthful and

Table 6.1: Comparison of Hormone Replacement Protocols

HORMONE	STANDARD MEDICAL PROTOCOL	DR. ULLIS PROTOCOL
Estrogen	Synthetic horse estrogen pills (Premarin)	Natural plant phytoestrogens Natural human bioidentical estrogen gel or cream
Progesterone	Synthetic Provera	Natural progesterone
Testosterone	None	DHEA Natural testosterone gel or cream

natural ratio. To give a woman estrogen alone will put her body in an unnatural and fattening hormonal imbalance.

One of the easiest and most natural ways to restore youthful testosterone levels is to go to your nearby health food store and buy the supplement dehydroepiandrosterone (DHEA), a naturally occurring human hormone that is a building block for your body to naturally produce testosterone. While DHEA is a weak testosterone booster for men, it is effective for menopausal women. Young women should not take DHEA or any other hormone supplement as it has adverse effects on reproduction. Small doses of DHEA (5 to 25 milligrams per day) are often enough to reliably increase women's testosterone to the levels that existed in their bodies when they were in their twenties. You will need to adjust your dose of DHEA to suit your needs: Start out with a low dose and increase it slowly until you feel rejuvenated and energized from achieving hormone balance.

Women on testosterone replacement therapy often report feeling youthful and rejuvenated, with more energy and sex drive than they ever had before. They also have much more energy and motivation for working out, and the fat and inches usually come off much more quickly. For some women, DHEA is not enough to bring about this hormone balance. If this is the case for you, talk to your doctor about taking prescription testosterone compounds in the form of gels or creams.

I have had tremendous success with my female patients with the use of testosterone replacement therapy. Whether a woman chooses DHEA or testosterone gels or creams, I always recommend medical supervision for any hormone replacement program. Testosterone in low doses is very safe and will do wonders for your diet and exercise program. But remember that hormones have powerful effects on your body, and it is always safest to have regular check-ups and to be in regular contact with a physician knowledgeable about hormone replacement therapy that involves the use of androgens.

Defeating Andropausal Weight Gain

As they get older, men suffer much of the same weight-gain problems as women do. The hormonal fat-burning advantage they have as young men slowly deteriorates with age. Some people also call this male equivalent of menopause "manopause," and a new scientific name for it is *male androgen insufficiency syndrome.* But it is most commonly called *andropause*, the term I will use to refer to this condition. The major difference between the two phenomena is that, whereas menopause hits women somewhat quickly and abruptly, andropause is often a slow and painful process.

Following the Hormone Revolution Weight-Loss Plan for proper diet, exercise, and supplements can help fight the hormonal imbalances associated with andropause. Generally, for three to six months andropausal men will make normal, steady progess in terms of losing fat and gaining muscle while on the program. Then some men will hit a rock-solid plateau and need stronger medicines to fight andropause.

The reason behind this plateau is the decline in testosterone levels in the aging man's body. This decline, which can start as early as age twenty-five or younger, gives them a huge disadvantage in burning fat and gaining muscle. To make things worse, estrogen levels can actually increase dramatically with age as the male body starts converting testosterone to estrogen. This combination of low testosterone and high estrogen during andropause can be disastrous to any weight-loss program and may even require medical therapies for many men.

Symptoms and Diagnosis of Andropause

For women, it is very easy to tell they are in menopause because of obvious signs such as a lack of menstrual periods and hot flashes. But, for men, this is not the case. Andropause comes on very slowly, so most men don't even know they have it. The first step toward fighting andropause is determining that you have it. Unfortunately, many of the symptoms of andropause are simply dismissed as inevitable and untreatable consequences of aging:

- loss of libido
- loss of sexual interest
- decrease in occurrence of morning erections
- fatigue
- depression
- irritability/edginess
- decrease in height
- penis/testicle shrinkage
- low self-esteem
- inability to lose fat
- inability to gain muscle

If you suffer from any of these symptoms, you should consult with your physician and have your blood tested for sex hormone imbalances before discussing treatment options. While estrogen and progesterone have been given to women for years to treat menopause, hormone replacement therapy for men has been quite rare until recently. Unfortunately, the medical establishment has been quite hostile to the idea of giving testosterone or other hormones to aging men, but this has all been slowly changing, and there are many options for boosting testosterone in andropausal men.

Arimidex: The MVP of Fighting Andropause

Arimidex (anastrozole) is one of the most effective choices for fighting the adverse symptoms of andropause, such as fatigue, lowered libido, depression, and weight gain. This is a drug approved by the FDA for treating breast cancer in women, but I have been a pioneer in its use as a hormone balancer for men. Arimidex is a highly safe and effective drug that stops the process in your body that converts testosterone into estrogen and sets off a series of reactions in the brain that signals it to produce more testosterone. It is extremely potent and in some cases restores a youthful testosterone/estrogen ratio in a matter of weeks.

The major drawback to Arimidex is the price, and it may not be covered by insurance as it is primarily a breast cancer medication. Its potency partially solves that problem because it is extremely effective in very low doses. Taking excessive doses of Arimidex can lower your estrogen too much, which can decrease your bone density and HDL cholesterol levels (good cholesterol), reduce your sex drive, and cause depression, among other side effects. Arimidex should be taken in very small doses, and those who take it should be closely monitored by their physicians. The FDA also has recently approved two new drugs that are similar to Arimidex: Femara (letrozole) and Aromasin (exemestane), which are also drugs that prevent the conversion of testosterone to estrogen. These new drugs may turn out to be more cost effective than Arimidex, although more research needs to be done.

Testosterone Replacement Therapy

For some men Arimidex is not enough to combat andropause, and they may require some other method of increasing testosterone. Testosterone has been falsely accused of being a dangerous anabolic steroid that causes overly aggressive behavior, and only recently has testosterone replacement or augmentation therapy become more widely accepted. Until recently, doctors across the country have been extremely reluctant to prescribe testosterone for anyone except those suffering from a severely debilitative condition, anemia, or other serious disease.

In the past, on the rare occasion when testosterone was prescribed, the therapy was incredibly inconvenient and required weekly injections. In addition, testosterone injections often produced either wildly fluctuating testosterone levels or very high levels, which caused natural testosterone production to shut down almost completely. Men on this old form of testosterone replacement therapy often experienced negative impacts on their mood, attitude, and sexuality as well. For many years, the only other alternatives for testosterone replacement therapy were various pills that contained testosterone or testosterone-like synthetic hormones that were often toxic to the liver and heart and only mildly effective at restoring youthful testosterone levels.

Fortunately for the andropausal men out there, the FDA has recently approved Androgel, a testosterone gel that can simply be rubbed on the skin every morning. No injections are required, and you don't have to take any pills. Androgel is very convenient to use, and studies have shown it to be extremely effective at boosting and maintaining testosterone levels without the likelihood of shutting down the body's testosterone production or causing liver toxicity. Androgel is remarkably effective for promoting success in men's diet and exercise programs, helping them both lose fat and gain muscle. Many men also experience a variety of other positive effects, such as increased energy, sex drive, erectile function, and improved mood.

Unlike Arimidex, Androgel is often covered by health insurance if a medical deficiency in testosterone can be established. The decision to use Arimidex, Androgel, or both is a personal choice that depends on my patients' medical profiles and lifestyle desires.

Other Treatments

The over-the-counter prohormone supplements mentioned in Chapter 4 can be used in cycles during andropause to get brief "pulses" of testosterone before sex or exercise. In particular, 100 to 200 milligrams of oral Androdiol (4-androstenediol) pills or 25 milligrams of sublingual Androdiol two or three times a week can give andropausal men an extra boost. It is also very important that andropausal men get enough zinc in their diets or take a multimineral with adequate zinc, as it plays an important role in preventing the conversion of testosterone to estrogen.

Human growth hormone (hGH) can be a powerful weapon against aging and andropause for a select few men. When combined with testosterone, hGH can have even more potent effects, but it requires expensive and inconvenient daily injections. Until more practical options are available, this therapy should be considered only for men with actual hGH deficiencies.

Safety of Testosterone

In general, you should feel quite safe and comfortable about boosting your testosterone levels with Arimidex, Androgel, or over-the-counter prohormones. But hormones are powerful tools, and they need to be administered carefully.

In the past, testosterone has been blamed for causing prostate problems, such as prostate cancer or benign prostate hypertrophy (BPH, or prostate enlargement), but it has never been shown or proven that testosterone causes prostate cancer. More recent research has suggested that estrogen may in fact be the bigger culprit in causing prostate problems and that maintaining a youthful testosterone/estrogen ratio may in fact prevent prostate problems. But still, it is better to be safe. I recommend that all men over the age of forty-five get tested regularly for prostate problems, whether or not they are on testosterone replacement therapy. Make sure your doctor gives you regular tests for prostate cancer and BPH, including measuring your blood levels of prostate specific antigen and giving you digital rectal examinations on a regular basis.

Testosterone also has been blamed for increasing the risk of heart disease. But recent research has shown that testosterone may actually lower the risk of heart disease for some men. Testosterone has been proven quite conclusively to be effective for helping you burn fat and gain muscle, and it is especially effective at burning abdominal fat. It also lowers insulin and LDL cholesterol levels in many men, melting their fat away. Anything that makes you leaner and more fit will likely decrease your risk of heart disease as well.

Don't just accept aging and andropause as an act of nature or God's natural intention. Far too many men simply "give up" as they get older. In the past, there really was not as much hope as there is now. Testosterone had a "big bad" stigma in the past, and most doctors were too scared or ignorant to do anything to help fight andropause. Now we have a full spectrum of options to help fight andropause and the obesity associated with it. Don't be afraid to ask your doctor about the various options available to you. Arimidex, Androgel, and other treatment options can jump-start your Hormone Revolution program.

SEVEN

LIFELONG BENEFITS

Losing weight and fat is just one of the numerous benefits of following the Hormone Revolution Weight-Loss Plan. Many aspects of this program will help fight and prevent diseases, enhance your sexuality both through a healthier libido as well as improved sexual function, and promote longevity. This chapter will explain how weight loss supported by a healthy hormone balance will improve your overall quality of life.

FIGHTING DISEASE

Some of the most frequently asked questions about the Hormone Revolution program are "Is it safe?" and "Does it have any side effects?" My answer to these questions is a resounding "yes." While conquering obesity on the Hormone Revolution program, you will experience side effects that include a lowered risk of many serious illnesses such as heart and cardiovascular disease, and increased immunity to common ailments such as colds and flus. The leanness and fitness you achieve through this program will bring you a higher level of overall health and physical well-being.

Modern medical science has found many advanced and expensive new techniques for diagnosing and treating all sorts of deadly diseases. But the simplest and cheapest way to treat many diseases is to prevent yourself from getting them in the first place. Unfortunately, there is no medical invention yet that will make you follow a healthy lifestyle that includes an appropriate and effective exercise and diet program. Until then, motivate yourself the best you can to stay with the Hormone Revolution program!

Heart and Cardiovascular Diseases

One of the most frequently used markers of heart health traditionally has been your total cholesterol level. Your total cholesterol number can be misleading, however, as there are two main types of cholesterol: LDL (bad cholesterol) and HDL (good cholesterol). The advanced medical circle is currently looking at cholesterol a bit differently by comparing the ratio of HDL cholesterol to LDL cholesterol. Based on this standard, an ideal diet program should be one that reduces your LDL cholesterol levels and increases your HDL cholesterol levels.

Unfortunately, many popular diets are clearly inappropriate for fighting heart disease because they do not take this ratio into consideration. Some of the popular low-carbohydrate diets can raise both your LDL and HDL cholesterol levels because of the large amount of saturated fats they allow, which raise your LDL levels. Any positive effects of increasing your good cholesterol levels are canceled out by the negative effects of increased bad cholesterol levels. Extremely low-fat diets have the opposite effect. If you follow one of these diets, your bad cholesterol levels will definitely drop. But the lack of fat in your diet will cause your good cholesterol levels to drop as well, causing you to simply break even when it comes to heart and cardiovascular health instead of improving it.

The emphasis in the Hormone Revolution Eating Plan (see Chapter 3) on healthy fats such as monounsaturated fats and omega-3 fatty acids will decrease bad cholesterol levels while simultaneously increasing good cholesterol levels. These effects are compounded by the exercise plan in Chapter 2, as the combination of aerobics and weight training will also strengthen your heart and circulatory system and decrease most risk factors for heart attacks and stroke.

Osteoporosis

Osteoporosis is a serious problem for many postmenopausal women as well as a significant risk for men over the age of sixty-five (most men are unfortunately ignorant of this risk). The drop in muscle and bone-building hormones (the same hormones that help you burn fat) with aging leads to loss of bone coupled with weight gain. Osteoporosis advances not only because of aging and loss of hormones but also because of inactivity, ill health, and certain medications. With all these factors taken together, the burden on your weakened bones becomes greater and greater, and your risk of serious fractures increases dramatically. The lack of mobility and the pain associated with osteoporotic fractures (especially hip fractures) can make life very miserable for many people and can lead to disability and even premature death.

Unfortunately, dieting can make osteoporosis worse. Improper dieting and exercising will lead not only to muscle loss but also to bone loss. To maintain or increase bone mass, you need to have an optimal balance of muscle- and bone-building hormones. Most diet plans will sabotage these hormones, causing major losses of bone mass and contributing to other factors that increase the risk of fractures.

The same hormones that are optimized to burn fat and build muscle will also increase bone mass and decrease your risk of osteoporosis. Only a diet that takes these powerful hormones into account will also help you to lose weight and fat without losing bone mass.

Cancer

Hormone balancing is very important for fighting many different types of cancer. For example, prostate cancer develops in many older men whose testosterone levels have dropped and estrogen levels increased. An excess of the wrong types of estrogens and insufficiencies of androgens (such as testosterone and DHEA) in women's bodies can eventually lead to breast cancer. But, by maintaining a youthful balance of testosterone, estrogen, and other hormones, men and women can greatly decrease their risk of these cancers.

Many food and supplement choices in the Hormone Revolution program help maintain these cancer-fighting hormone balances. Unprocessed fruits and vegetables contain not only essential vitamins, minerals, and fiber but also naturally occurring compounds such as valuable plant pigments and *phytonutrients* (plant nutrients). Phytonutrients and plant pigments play a protective role for the human body, helping to protect it against cancer (particularly of the breast and prostate) and other diseases.

Diabetes

Poor dietary and lifestyle choices and other factors have lead to a rapid increase in the rate of diabetes in the United States. Almost every step in the Hormone Revolution program will help prevent diabetes and relieve the stress on the insulin system from those already suffering from the disease. A diet rich in healthy fats and high-fiber colored vegetables is excellent for balancing your body's blood sugar and insulin levels. Eating smaller meals throughout the day instead of one or two big meals will also help improve your body's insulin function, as will aerobic and weight-bearing exercise. Most important, losing weight and fat is also one of the best ways to improve your insulin function and prevent diabetes.

Colds and Flus

Many diets that lead to starvation and overtraining can wreak havoc within your immune system and cause many people to catch colds and flus more frequently. The Hormone Revolution Program protects your immune system in several key ways. The healthy sources of protein, fats, and phytonutrients recommended in this book, along with the core supplement program and moderate exercise, can give your immune system a tremendous boost. Essential vitamins and minerals are necessary for a strong immune response to all the bugs and viruses we are exposed to daily. The allergic responses that often lead to chronic infections such as bronchitis and sinusitis can be reduced. Many studies have shown that zinc, vitamin C, and antioxidant nutrients may help prevent colds and flus as well as shorten the duration of these illnesses.

Memory Impairment

As we age, many of our cognitive functions decline. Most people eventually succumb to age-associated memory impairment (AAMI), a slow and subtle decline in memory that occurs in aging people. Extreme cases result in Alzheimer's disease, a serious condition that involves significant declines in our capacity to carry out almost all daily life functions. Loss of memory is a problem even for young people, and losing the ability to remember, concentrate, and focus also greatly detracts from your enjoyment of life. Diets that lead to starvation are especially likely to make it more difficult for you to concentrate and focus on your life's daily tasks.

To combat this, the Hormone Revolution Eating Plan includes monounsaturated fats, which not only protect against heart disease but also guard against mental decline and improve brain-cell functioning. There is also evidence that the hormone-balancing antioxidants and pigments derived from eating fruits and vegetables and from taking supplements also improve brain function. Hormonal imbalances have been linked to Alzheimer's disease and to other neurological impairments. In fact, recent research has suggested that testosterone, antioxidants, and vitamins C and E may help prevent Alzheimer's disease. While more research needs to be done, I believe that the combination of appropriate exercise, antioxidant supplements, hormone balancing, and a diet rich in colored fruits and vegetables will reduce your risk of getting Alzheimer's disease and other brain disorders associated with aging.

Chronic Fatigue

Chronic fatigue is not medically considered or classified as a disease, which is unfortunate considering the great degree to which it affects so many people, especially those over forty. Fatigue is often a symptom of accelerated aging, hormone imbalances, poor eating habits, and improper exercising. Fatigue and weight loss go hand in hand. Many people say they are highly motivated to begin a diet and exercise program but simply lack the energy because of overwhelming chronic fatigue. Even younger people suffer from fatigue because of overtraining and improper exercising. By addressing the problems of aging, hormone imbalances, and appropriate diet and exercise, the Hormone Revolution Weight-Loss Plan eliminates the burden of fatigue.

Depression

Obesity and depression go hand in hand. Depression often leads to excessive eating and thus obesity, and obesity is often a major source or symptom of depression. Sometimes it is hard to know which comes first, the disturbed eating or the depression. Any program that fights abnormal eating patterns and obesity also will improve symptoms of depression.

Depressed people often seek comfort and relief from anxiety in food, especially sugars and starches. What they do not realize is that the brain is asking for signal balancing, and consuming sugar and starches, along with fats, is how many people self-medicate their mood imbalances. But this is only a temporary solution, which can be corrected in the long term by hormone balance induced through proper diet and exhilarating exercise.

SEX AND VITALITY

A telltale symptom of an improper diet and exercise plan is a loss of sexual interest, function, and pleasure. Far too many people simply give up and think that getting fatter and losing their sex lives is an inevitable fact of aging. And many others let obesity stand in their way of pleasurable sex lives. But maintaining or restoring a youthful balance of hormones not only can accelerate fat burning and weight loss but also can greatly enhance sexual interest and performance.

Sex and Weight Loss: The Intimate Connection

There is a very strong connection between weight loss and sex drive. The hormones you stimulate during exercise directly turn on your body's natural fat-burning and muscle-building mechanisms and change your behavior and attitude, increasing your libido in the process. And good sex is an excellent exercise that helps burn calories. Since a greater libido usually means having more sex, boosting your libido usually means getting leaner.

Another thing to keep in mind is that getting leaner and boosting your libido will help your spouse or partner lose weight. Hormonal weight loss is contagious and can be caught by those you are intimate with. This happens because your fat-burning hormone levels will go up when you are sexually aroused. If you become lean and fit and more attractive to your spouse or partner, he or she, in turn, will become more aroused and also experience a fat-burning hormonal boost. The motivation to exercise and have more sex also will increase. This is one reason why I often encourage people to begin their Hormone Revolution with the partners they love.

Sex as a Measure of Progress

Pay close attention to the level and degree of your sexual thoughts and fantasies when you start dieting or exercising. These can serve as excellent measures of the effectiveness of your program. If your sexual interest increases, you are likely doing everything right, but if you notice a drop in your sex drive while on a diet and exercise program, you need to adjust your program. Libido is an excellent and very strong marker of a proper hormonal balance. If your libido actually drops, it means you are wreaking havoc on your hormonal system through overtraining or starvation. Even teenagers or people in their twenties frequently notice a loss of libido when they diet or exercise in an improper way.

If you follow my program closely, you should experience an increase in libido within two to three weeks. In the rare case that your libido doesn't increase or even drops a little bit, look carefully at your diet and exercise logs. Try easing up a bit on your aerobics and adding an extra-small meal or snack every day. Also, it is especially important to have your Magic Window Meal after every workout.

Some of the people who follow my program for a long time generally experience a greater libido at first but after four to six months feel a drop. In these rare cases, I recommend that they stop exercising for one to two weeks. Low libido may be a sign that the body needs a short break, perhaps a vacation away from home that does not involve intense physical or mental activity. Your libido should come back stronger than ever after a nice break.

Sleep and Relaxation

As mentioned before, proper sleep and relaxation are essential to the Hormone Revolution program. Deep and continuous sleep is essential for building and repairing muscles and other body tissues. Lack of relaxation and out-of-control stress also throw your hormones out of balance and can lead to fat gain and muscle loss.

Mutually good sex with a partner is a proven method for decreasing mental stress and often helps you get better sleep. The increased libido and sex drive generated by this program should greatly assist you in these areas. Remember that while you are enjoying your sex life, you also are greatly assisting your Hormone Revolution program.

LIVING LEAN, LIVING LONG

The most proven and widely researched method of extending life is caloric restriction. It has been well demonstrated in many species, from insects to mice, rats, and monkeys. There is a growing consensus among doctors and scientists that eating fewer calories along with optimizing nutrition will add many good-quality years to your life. A diet and exercise program such as this one that leads to long-term caloric restriction also will work as an effective life-extension plan.

Most life-extension plans say nothing about enhancing the pleasures of life while living longer. Spending your life constantly starving or craving foods is no way to live life happily. Therefore, the Hormone Revolution definition of life extension does not just mean staying alive, but extending and increasing your capacity to actually enjoy your life by improving your body's functions.

Dieting Without Starvation

The Hormone Revolution Eating Plan allows for eating a wide variety of foods at appropriate times throughout the day. Instead of ignoring the cravings for the foods many people enjoy, this program shows you how to harness these cravings into an effective eating plan that will stimulate your fat-burning hormones and control your appetite. Eating a wide spectrum of foods will keep your appetite under control while enabling you to enjoy the foods you love.

Happiness and Fat Loss

While having to support excess pounds is physically hard on your body, it is even harsher on your emotional and personal life. Obesity can lead to loss of self-esteem, depression, emotional fatigue, and job and relationship problems. While there is a recent movement accusing those who want to be lean and fit of vanity, the truth is that conquering obesity is often a matter of profound psychological significance. Becoming attractive to yourself and to others is essential to self-esteem and emotional well-being and perhaps even to your financial well-being and professional success.

Extending Human Limits

Another important aspect of life extension is overcoming personal physical limitations. For many people, obesity limits their ability to perform even trivial daily activities, such as moving efficiently or tying their own shoes, impairing their capacity to enjoy life on the most basic level. In severe cases, some become too obese to walk and are bedridden.

But the stronger and more mobile you are, the greater your capacity to enjoy life. The Hormone Revolution Weight-Loss Plan is intended not to be simply cosmetic but instead to afford people the basic fitness required to maintain a strength of body to carry out life's functions energetically and enthusiastically. The program emphasizes standing free-weight exercises not only because these exercises build muscle but also because the strength they impart makes it easier to cope with life's physical requirements such as lifting and bending. A positive side effect of this body conditioning is that you also will look and feel youthful and fit.

A Sustainable Life-Extension Plan

The challenge in developing my Hormone Revolution program was not choosing the right foods to eat or the right exercises to do. Rather, the biggest challenge for me was finding a program that could be easily maintained by the average person with a family, a busy work schedule, and financial constraints.

Most of us don't have enough time or money to devote our lives to physical fitness and staying lean. Obligations to our family, friends, and jobs are always our high priorities. But the Hormone Revolution program is designed to save time so that you can fit it into your everyday schedule as easily as possible. Having more energy and greater physical capacity makes you more productive and efficient and allows you more time to enjoy yourself.

I hope this book has helped you to understand the important impact that hormones have on your weight-loss goals and on so many other aspects of your life. I have worked to develop a program that any person, regardless of age or gender, can follow and sustain for a lifetime to achieve the lasting benefits of hormonal balance and fitness. So get started, stick with it, and join the Hormone Revolution!

CREATING
A PERSONALIZED PROGRAM

I originally developed this program while working one on one with patients in my own clinic, where I was able to address their individual needs and assess their progress. My goal in this book was to include this personal advice and to condense vast amounts of information into an inclusive and comprehensive program. But many aspects of the program still require interaction with health care and fitness professionals. Although I cannot provide this service to all of my readers, I would like to supply them with an ongoing, interactive resource. So I invite all of you who seek more detailed information about the Hormone Revolution Weight-Loss Plan to visit my website at www.HormoneRevolution.com.

I developed this website to better assist my patients and readers in keeping up to date on the latest research on weight loss, antiaging medicine, and general health and fitness. On it, you will find information about how you can customize your Hormone Revolution program according to age, gender, lifestyle, hormonal profiles, and many other factors. I also have a section where the most frequently asked questions about the Hormone Revolution program are answered and additional fitness and diet tips are offered. You can post messages and exchange ideas with others who have discovered the Hormone Revolution.

Karlis Ullis, M.D., can be reached at
KUllis@HormoneRevolution.com or
Sports Medicine and Anti-Aging Medical Group
1807 Wilshire Boulevard, Suite #205
Santa Monica, CA 90403
(310) 829-1990
Fax: (310) 829-5134

Joshua Shackman, Ph.D., can be reached at
JShackman@HormoneRevolution.com

APPENDIX I:
BASIC EXERCISE INSTRUCTIONS

WEIGHT-LIFTING INSTRUCTIONS

I really wish I could teach you all the finer points of weight training through this book, but it is impossible to learn without personal training from a professional. But I do think it is useful to take a look at what weight-training exercises I recommend the most and to get an idea of how to do them. The information presented here is intended to give you a general idea of how to exercise correctly with weights. Make sure you go through all these exercises first with a personal trainer or experienced health care professional. Do not try to do these on your own first, especially if you have never lifted weights before or have not lifted for over one year.

For each exercise in this appendix, do an easy warm-up set of 8 to 10 repetitions. Then do 8 to 10 repetitions of heavier weights. The last 2 or 3 reps should be difficult, and you should feel like your muscles are maxed out: They should hit muscle failure—the point where your muscles cannot contract anymore. If you feel more than just regular muscle soreness, *stop right away* to avoid injury, and get advice.

Upper-Body Exercises

Both men and women must do a variety of upper-body exercises. Women often neglect these exercises for fear of becoming overly muscular. But it is important to work out the major muscle groups in the upper body regardless of gender. This is essential for stimulating your fat-burning hormones and for maintaining strength and muscle mass while losing weight. As mentioned before, most women will not get overly muscular from doing upper-body exercises.

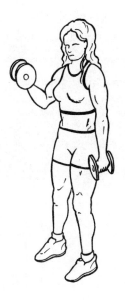

1. Standing Biceps Dumbbell Curls

• Put a single-weight dumbbell in each hand. While keeping your elbow still at your side, lift the weight upward toward your chest with your left arm and then return it to your side. Repeat, using your right arm. Alternate lifts with right arm and left arm.

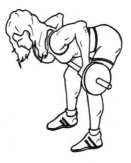

2. Bent-Over Rows

• Bend over as pictured in the illustration above. Bend your knees about 20 to 40 degrees and lower the weight bar until your arms are extended fully. Stay bent forward at the waist to about 20 to 40 degrees above the plane of the floor. Keep your bend at an angle that feels comfortable on the lower back. Now lift the bar up toward the lower chest and squeeze the shoulder blades together as you lift the weight toward the chest. You should maintain a small natural curve in the back while doing this exercise.

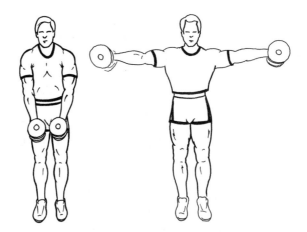

3. Lateral Raises

• Start with a dumbbell in each hand at your side, with your elbows extended straight while standing up straight. Now raise the weights out from your sides to an angle that is parallel with the floor, so that your arms are perpendicular to your body.

• Slowly and gradually bring the weights back to your sides and repeat.

• Caution: If you have shoulder problems, do not raise the weights higher than what feels comfortable or up to shoulder level. This is to avoid compression of the supra spinatous and rotator cuff tendons of the shoulder.

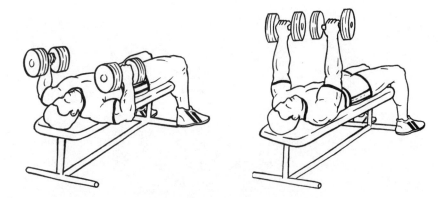

4. Dumbbell Bench Press

• Lie face up on a bench with legs flat on the ground or flat on the bench and with a dumbbell in each hand that has the ends aligned with the length of your body.

• Keep your upper arms parallel with the floor, so that your elbows are slightly above your chest. Slowly bring the dumbbells up so that the ends touch at the end in front of you. Then slowly and gradually return to the start position.

• Caution: Do not let the elbows drop below chest level. If you have shoulder problems, then keep the elbows above the plane of the floor and do shorter arc presses upward.

Lower-Body Exercises

Far too many men ignore lower-body exercises altogether and only focus on the upper body. This is a huge mistake. It is very important to work out the lower body, as it includes some of the largest muscle groups in your body. You are getting only half the effects of weight training if you only exercise your upper body.

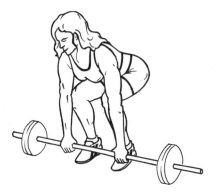

1. Bent-Leg Dead Lifts

• These are very powerful lifts that stimulate large amounts of muscle all at once. Reach over to pick up the weight with your knees bent as in the illustration above. Be sure to bend your knees and keep your back almost flat except for a small natural curve at the lower back. Just lift the weight by going from a squatting to a standing position using the power of your legs.

• Note: Straight-leg dead lifts are okay if you have a strong back. Go easy with this one and slowly build up. Be very careful if you have back problems.

2. High Pulls

• Begin slightly bent over with your legs straight. Hold a barbell at knee height. Pull up the barbell as high as you can to chest level or to the nipple line. Do what feels most comfortable at first.

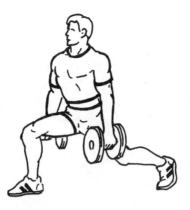

3. Lunge Squats or Lunge Walking

• Spread your legs in a walking position with a large stride as in the illustration above, with a barbell in each hand. Move your legs to a standing position while keeping your back straight.

• These are great for working the leg muscles. You may want to begin with plain squats without any lunges at all when first starting your program. Do a dry run without weights first if you are a beginner or have knee or lower-extremity problems. If you are okay with that, then do some lunge squatting or walking holding a dumbbell in each hand.

• In general, do not squat at an angle of the thigh to the leg that is greater than 90 degrees. If you have knee problems, then do "partial squats" or just squat to a level that feels comfortable.

Abdominal Muscle Exercises

You must work *all the abdominal muscle groups.* The abdominal muscles are complex and consist of the upper and lower abdominals and the *obliques,* the abdominals at the sides. A common misconception of many people is that by doing "crunches" they have worked all the abs and that's all that's required. Later they wonder why their tummies are not perfectly flat or don't look like "six packs." Doing generic crunches only works one portion of the four major abdominal groups.

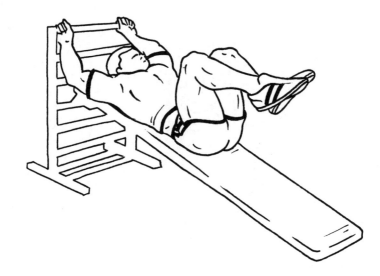

1. Reverse Crunches

- A reverse crunch works the lower abs.
- Lie down on your back. You can do this using a bench or the floor as the exercise platform.
- Breathe out as you raise the knees and legs up toward your belly button. Keep the back flat against the ground or bench. Keep the neck relaxed.
- When your abs get stronger, you can use an adjustable bench and tilt the bench in a downward slope so that you are lifting more of the lower part of the body upward against gravity. Hold on to the bench with your hands over your head or at the sides when doing incline reverse crunches.

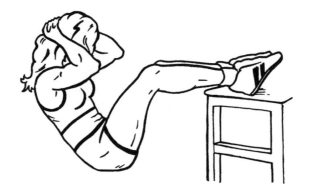

2. Traditional Ab Crunches *(see bottom page 164)*

• Put the back of your legs flat on top of a chair so you have a 90-degree angle between the thigh and leg. Tuck your chin in toward the chest and support your neck by locking your fingers behind the neck and keeping the elbows parallel. Keep the neck still and relaxed and supported by your interlocked fingers.

• Lift the shoulders and chest above the ground. Be careful not to move your chin or neck about, since this may produce undue neck strain. Your neck should not feel strained if properly supported by your locked hands and fingers. You should feel tightness-contraction in the upper abdomen. When you are stronger and if you do not have a back problem, then try to go all the way up, almost touching the elbows to the knees.

• To work the "side abs," come up and turn, slightly pointing one elbow toward the opposite knee. Come back down and alternate the motion toward the opposite knee.

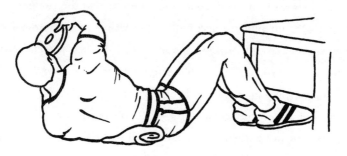

3. Lateral Twists–Lateral Ab Exercises

Once you have gotten stronger at the abs with the other two ab exercises you may want to add the advanced lateral twists that exercise the oblique (side) abdominal muscles. These are often neglected by most people who exercise. This will require a lot of coordination and balance and works many muscles at once.

• Get a weight plate of 1 to 5 pounds. Lie back with a small towel. Roll in the small of your back. Hold the plate in front of you and come up holding it away from the body with the arms straight at the elbows.

• Your back should be at about a 30- to 40-degree angle to the floor. Once you are stable, then, while keeping the arms out straight, rotate/twist to the left while keeping the right lower back on the towel. Go as far as comfortable, then come back to the center and repeat. Take a break. Then repeat the same with a twist to the right side. A medicine ball also can serve the same purpose as a weight plate.

• I personally prefer a medicine ball for my own lateral twist exercise workouts. It is easy to hold a small medicine ball. This exercise will tighten your neck muscles. If you have a neck problem, go slow and use a lighter weight. Do it under supervision or avoid this exercise.

• My own neck occasionally hurts. After slowly building up using this lateral twist exercise, I have been able to strengthen my neck and feel better overall. It is a powerful trunk and ab exercise.

Part of the reason for weak abdominal muscles and the "bulging gut" is that we all sit a lot plus we accumulate fat within the abdominal cavity. While we sit, the "ab" muscles go slack and get weak. I recommend that during sitting at work you do some "ab" exercises daily.

While sitting at your chair, hold your back straight and extend your legs and alternate a scissors motion with the legs or do a pedaling motion by raising and lowering one leg at a time without letting the legs touch the ground.

You also can hold both legs/knees together and raise them together straight upward toward the belly button—a reverse crunch. You should be able to feel contractions (tightness in the lower abdominal muscles). By turning the legs to the right of center and lifting them up toward you and then to the left you will work both the side and lower abs.

APPENDIX II:

INFORMATION RESOURCES

AgingPrevent.com
or HormoneRevolution.com

Official webpage for Karlis Ullis, M.D. Includes updates and the latest information on the Hormone Revolution Weight-Loss Plan as well as information on how to join the exclusive Longevity Rx Group (an Internet and in-person private discussion group).

Cognitive Enhancement Research Institute
www.ceri.com
P.O. Box 4029
Menlo Park, CA 94026
USA
650-321-CERI (650-321-2374)

The institute is dedicated to promoting longevity and antiaging medicine, with an emphasis on cognitive enhancement and brain longevity. Has a referral list of physicians, many of whom are knowledgeable about anti-aging medicine and hormone replacement therapy. Also includes a listing of pharmacies that specially compound natural hormone replacement creams and gels.

Dr. Squat
www.drsquat.com

A webpage devoted to information about weight training that was created by Dr. Frederick Hatfield. Publishes the "Iron Web" newsletter and has a lot of useful information on exercises using free weights while standing. Dr. Frederick Hatfield is also the president and cofounder of the International Sports Sciences Association (www.issaonline.com). The ISSA publishes the book *Fitness, The Complete Guide,* which contains much information on weight training and general health and fitness.

Life Extension Foundation
www.lef.org
1100 W. Commercial Boulevard
Fort Lauderdale, FL 33309
(800) 544-4440

This organization is dedicated to promoting life-extension research and education. Publishes a monthly magazine and has a large archive of articles and information on its website.

Los Angeles Gerontology Research Group
www.grg.org

This group of doctors and scientists studies research on life extension and antiaging medicine. Founded by leading gerontology researcher Stephen Coles, M.D., Ph.D.

Muscle Monthly
www.MuscleMonthly.com

A scientifically oriented fitness magazine, with articles written by leading health and fitness experts. Website has an archive of articles from the authors of this publication. Also has an on-line supplement store.

The Supplement Research Foundation
www.tsrf.com

Foundation dedicated to promoting research and education in the area of dietary supplements. Founded by leading supplement and nutrition expert Rehan Jalali, B.S.

Think Muscle Magazine
www.thinkmuscle.com

On-line health and fitness magazine dedicated to providing its readers with the latest scientific research on diet, nutrition, and supplements. Includes an archive of articles from the authors of this publication.

Tourou University International (TUI)
College of Health Sciences
http://www.tourou.edu/HSM.htm
infochs@tourou.
5665 Plaza Drive, 3rd Floor
Cypress, CA 90630

Listed by *U.S. News & World Report* as one of the nation's best on-line graduate programs, TUI's College of Health Sciences offers a wide variety of on-line courses in nutrition and other health and fitness-related topics taught by leading experts in the field. These classes can be applied to a fully accredited B.S., M.S., or Ph.D. in Health Sciences as well as to a variety of certificate programs.

Creative Health Products
www.chponilne.com
5148 Saddle Ridge Road
Plymouth, MI 48170
(800) 742-4478
Fax: (734) 996-4650

Sells fitness products: monitoring devices, exercise equipment, calipers, step counters, digital pedometers, cardio trainers that combine heart rate with distance measurement—pedometers, BioImpedance body-fat analyzer scales: Tanita brands and software for newer Tanita scales and other brands of fat analyzers.

Digiwalker
www.digiwalker.com

Sells the Digiwalker device mentioned in this book.

Netrition.com

Sells a wide assortment of supplements, books, and food products. Includes a "Very Low-Carb Products" section that includes high-protein designer foods compatible with the "Standard Meals" included in the Hormone Revolution Weight-Loss Plan.

Tanita Corporation of America
www.tanita.com

Tanita is the manufacturer of home body-fat scales. The website has information on various models, as well as a listing of stores that sell the scales.

SUPPLEMENT RESOURCES

Note: These are companies that patients of Karlis Ullis, M.D., have found to be reliable in terms of quality. Listing here does not necessarily imply an endorsement.

PART I

Companies that sell supplements only on the recommendation of a health care professional. The supplements that are provided by these companies are not available over the counter.

Designs for Health Institute, Inc.
2 North Road
Windsor, CT 06088
(800) 847-8302
www.designsforhealth.com

Has l-carnitine powder and caps, phosphatidyl serine powder, and other useful powder and capsule formulations for weight and fat loss and for regulating metabolism. Also offers advanced seminars in clinical nutrition for health care practitioners.

Integrative Therapeutics (IT), Inc.
9725 S.W. Commerce Circle
Suite A6
Wilsonville, OR 97070
(800) 931-1709
Local: (503) 582-8386

Fax: (503) 582-0386

e-mail: Info@integrativeinc.com

Integrative Therapeutics (IT), Inc., is a partnership of providers of nutritional supplements that includes PhytoPharmacia of Green Bay, Wisconsin, and NF Formulas, Tyler Encapsulations, and Vitaline Formulas of Wilsonville, Oregon. The Tyler formulations are usually available only on the recommendation of a health care practitioner. Some of the other mentioned brands are available over the counter.

Metagenics

100 Avenida La Pata

San Clemente, CA 92673

(800) 692-9400

www.metagenics.com

Sells a full line of supplements.

Tyler Encapsulations

9725 S.W. Commerce Circle

Wilsonville, OR 97070

(800) 869-9705

www.tyler-inc.com

Sells high-grade supplements.

PART II

Supplement companies that sell on an over-the-counter basis. Supplements sold by the companies below are sold directly to consumers at health food and sports nutrition stores as well as over the Internet.

Ergopharm
205 S. Main
P.O. Box 160
Seymour, IL 61875
Fax: (217) 687-4138
www.ergopharm.net

Supplement company specializing in prohormone products, including Androdiol and the new prohormone 1AD. Also offers a thermogenic product.

Prolab
(800) 776-6177
e-mail: CUSTOMERSERVICE@PROLAB.com
http://www.prolab.com/

Has an extensive line of diet and sports nutrition products, many of which are compatible with the Hormone Revolution Weight-Loss Plan. Its parent company, Natrol (www.Natrol.com), also sells high-quality supplements, including many of those mentioned in this book.

Super Nutrition
Oakland, CA 94612
(800) 262-2116
www.supernutritionusa.com

Has many vitamin, mineral, antioxidant, and phytonutrient blends; available at many retail outlets.

APPENDIX III:

EXPERTISE

Anna Brantman, M.S.

Nutritional Director, Hormone Revolution Weight-Loss Plan

Nutritional Director, Sports Medicine and Anti-Aging Medical Group

1807 Wilshire Boulevard, Suite # 205

Santa Monica, CA 90403

(310) 829-1990

Fax: (310) 829-5134

e-mail: integrative1@hotmail.com

Robert Crayhon, M.S., C.N.

Designs for Health Institute

5345 Arapahoe #3

Boulder, CO 80303

(303) 415-0229

www.dfhi.com

Cory Everson
www.coryeverson.com

Cory Everson is a world-renowned health and fitness expert. She has several exercise books and videos, and is a respected fitness lecturer and television personality. She also is a six-time Ms. Olympia.

Dr. Frederick Hatfield
President and Cofounder, International Sports Sciences Association
www.drsquat.com
www.issaonline.com

Dr. Hatfield (a.k.a. Dr. Squat) is a well-known training consultant to professional sports teams, sports governing bodies, and world-class and professional athletes. He has a great deal of experience in academia, powerlifting, and the fitness industry. Hatfield was inducted into the Powerlifting Hall of Fame in 2000 and holds numerous powerlifting records.

Institute for Functional Medicine (IFM)
P.O. Box 1729
Gig Harbor, WA 98335
(800) 843-9660; (253) 851-3943
www.functionalmedicine.org

Specializes in advanced professional nutritional seminars and functional food design.

Mason Panetti, Nutritional Counselor
e-mail: GuineaPigRx@netscape.net

Twelve years of experience in food-plan assembly, nutritional supplement counseling, and nutritional supplement research/development for average individuals, elite athletes, and model/actors.

Cristiana Paul, M.S. Nutrition Science
e-mail: CristianaP@aol.com

Diet and supplement plans for sports nutrition, antiaging, diabetes, and cardiovascular diseases.

Karlis Ullis, M.D.
Medical Director
Sports Medicine and Anti-Aging Medical Group
1807 Wilshire Boulevard, Suite # 205
Santa Monica, CA 90403
(310) 829-1990
Fax: (310) 829-5134

SELECTED REFERENCES

GENERAL

Chakravarthy, M.V.; Joyner, M.J.; and Booth, F.W. "An Obligation for Primary Care Physicians to Prescribe Physical Activity to Sedentary Patients to Reduce the Risk of Chronic Health Conditions." *Mayo Clinic Proceedings.* 2002 Feb; 77(2): 165–73. Review.

Holden, C. "Cracking the Secrets of Aging." *Science.* 2002 Feb 8; 295(5557): 1033.

Johnston, C.S.; Day, C.S.; and Swan, P.D. "Postprandial Thermogenesis Is Increased 100% on a High-Protein, Low-Fat Diet Versus a High-Carbohydrate, Low-Fat Diet in Healthy, Young Women." *Journal of the American College of Nutrition.* 2002 Feb; 21(1): 55–61.

Ludwig, D.S.; Pereira, M.A.; et al. "Dietary Fiber, Weight Gain and Cardiovascular Risk Factors in Young Adults." *Journal of the American Medical Association.* 1999 Oct 27; 282(16): 1539–1646.

Mokdad, A.H.; Bowman, B.A.; Ford, E.S.; et al. "The Continuing Epidemics of Obesity and Diabetes in the United States." *Journal of the American Medical Association.* 2001 Sept 12; 286(10): 1195–1200.

Nied, R.J.; and Franklin, B. "Promoting and Prescribing Exercise for the Elderly." *American Family Physician.* 2002 Feb 1; 65(3): 419–26.

The NutriBase Nutrition Facts Desk Reference. New York: Avery, 2001.

Ullis, Karlis; and Ptacek, Greg. *Age Right.* New York: Simon & Schuster, 1999.

Ullis, Karlis; Ptacek, Greg; and Shackman, Joshua. *Super "T."* New York: Fireside Books, a division of Simon & Schuster, 1999. Includes appendix from Cristiana Paul, M.S.

Urhausen, A.; and Kindermann, W. "Diagnosis of Overtraining: What Tools Do We Have?" *Sports Medicine.* 2002; 32(2): 95–102.

HORMONES AND BODY COMPOSITION

Anawalt, B.D.; et al. "Testosterone Administration to Normal Men Decreases Truncal and Total Body Fat." Presented at 1999 Endrocrine Society conference, San Diego, CA.

Blackman, M.R.; et al. "Effects of Growth Hormone and/or Sex Steroid Administration on Body Composition in Healthy Elderly Women and Men." Presented at 1999 Endrocrine Society conference, San Diego, CA.

Espeland, M.A.; et al. "Effect of Postmenopausal Hormone Therapy on Body Weight and Waist and Hip Girths." *Journal of Clinical Endocrinology and Metabolism.* 1997 May; 82(5): 1549–56.

Kaye, S.A.; et al. "Associations of Body Mass and Fat Distribution with Sex Hormone Concentrations in Postmenopausal Women." *Journal of Epidemiology.* 1991 Mar; 20(1): 151–6.

Lovejoy, et al. "Exogenous Androgens Influence Body Composition and Regional Body Fat Distribution in Obese Postmenopausal Women—A Clinical Research Center Study." *Journal of Clinical Endocrinology and Metabolism.* 1996 June; 81(6): 2198–2203.

O'Sullivan, A.J.; et al. "The Route of Estrogen Replacement Therapy Confers Divergent Effects on Substrate Oxidation and Body Composition in Postmenopausal Women." *Journal of Clinical Investigations.* 1998 Sept 1; 102(5): 1035–40.

Pasquali, R.; et al. "The Relative Contribution of Androgens and Insulin in Determining Abdominal Body Fat Distribution in Premenopausal Women." *Journal of Endocrinological Investigations.* 1991 Nov; 14(10): 839–46.

Stoll, B.A. "Perimenopausal Weight Gain and Progression of Breast Cancer Precursors." *Cancer Detection and Prevention.* 1999; 23(1): 31–36.

Yoo, K.Y.; et al. "Female Sex Hormones and Body Mass in Adolescent and Postmenopausal Korean Women." *Journal of Korean Medical Sciences.* 1998 June; 13(3): 241–6.

ESTROGEN REPLACEMENT THERAPY

Chen, Y.; Liu, X.; Pisha, E.; Constantinou, A.I.; Hua, Y.; Shen, L.; van Breemen, R.B.; Elguindi, E.C.; Blond, S.Y.; Zhang, F.; and Bolton, J.L. "Metabolite of Equine Estrogens, 4-hydroxyequilenin, Induces DNA Damage and Apoptosis in Breast Cancer Cell Lines." *Chemical Research in Toxicology.* 2000 May; 13(5): 342–50.

O'Sullivan, A.J.; Crampton, L.J.; Freund, J.; and Ho, K.K. "The Route of Estrogen Replacement Therapy Confers Divergent Effects on Substrate Oxidation and Body Composition in Postmenopausal Women." *Journal of Clinical Investigations.* 1998 Sept 1; 102(5): 1035–40.

Persson, I.; Thurfjell, E.; Bergstrom, R.; and Holmberg, L. "Hormone Replacement Therapy and the Risk of Breast Cancer. Nested Case-Control Study in a Cohort of Swedish Women Attending Mammography Screening." *International Journal of Cancer.* 1997 Sept 4; 72(5): 758–61.

SUPPLEMENTS

Astrup, Arne; et al. "Enhanced Thermogenic Responsiveness During Chronic Ephedrine Treatment in Man." *American Journal of Clinical Nutrition* 42(July 1985): 83–94.

Astrup, Arne; et al. "The Effect of Ephedrine/Caffeine Mixture on Energy Expenditure and Body Composition in Obese Woman." *Metabolism.* 1992; 1(7): 686–8.

Dulloo, A.G.; Duret, C.; Rohrer, D.; Girardier, L.; Mensi, N.; Fathi, M.; Chantre, P.; and Vandermander, J. "Efficacy of a Green Tea Extract Rich in Catechin Polyphenols and Caffeine in Increasing 24-h Energy Expenditure and Fat Oxidation in Humans." *American Journal of Clinical Nutrition.* 1999; 70(6): 1040–45.

Dulloo, A.G.; Seydoux, J.; Girardier, L.; Chantre, P.; and Vandermander, J. "Green Tea and Thermogenesis: Interactions Between Catechin-Polyphenols, Caffeine and Sympathetic Activity." *International Journal of Obesity and Related Metabolic Disorders.* 2000; 24(2): 252–58.

Earnest, C.; Snell, P.; Rodriguez, R.; Almada, A.; and Mitchell, T. "The Effect of Creatine Monohydrate Ingestion on Anaerobic Power Indices, Muscular Strength and Body Composition." *Acta Physiologica Scandinavica* 153(1995): 207–9.

Fahey, et al. "Hormonal Effects of Phosphatidylserine (PS) During Two Weeks of Intense Weight Training." Presented at 1998 ACSM conference, Orlando, FL.

Gordon, A.; Hultman, E.; Kaijser, L.; Kristgansson, S.; Rolf, C.; Nyquist, O.; et al. "Creatine Supplementation in Chronic Heart Failure Increases Skeletal Muscle Creatine Phosphate and Muscle Performance." *Cardiovascular Research* 30(1995): 413–18.

Jialal, I.; and Grundy, S. "Effect of Combined Supplementation with Alpha-Tocopherol, Ascorbate and Beta-Carotene on Low-Density Lipoprotein Oxidation." *Circulation* 88(1993): 2780–86.

Kreider, R.; Klesges, R.; Harmon, K.; Grindstaff, P.; Ramsey, L.; Bullen, D.; et al. "Effects of Ingesting Supplements Designed to Promote Lean Tissue Accretion on Body Composition During Resistance Exercise." *International Journal of Sport Nutrition* 6(1996): 234–46.

Monteleone, P.; Maj, M.; Beinat, L.; Natale, M.; and Kemali, D. "Blunting by Chronic Phosphatidylserine Administration of the Stress-Induced Activation of the Hypothalamo-Pituitary-Adrenal Axis in Healthy Men." *European Journal of Clinical Pharmacology.* 1992; 42(4): 385–88.

Mori, T.A.; Burke, V.; Puddey, I.B.; Watts, G.F.; O'Neal, D.N.; Best, J.D.; and Beilin, L.J. "Purified Eicosapentaenoic and Docosahexaenoic Acids Have Differential Effects on Serum Lipids and Lipoproteins, LDL Particle Size, Glucose, and Insulin in Mildly Hyperlipidemic Men." *American Journal of Clinical Nutrition* 71(2000): 1085–94.

Pasquali, Renato; et al. "Effects of Chronic Administration of Ephedrine During Very-Low-Calorie Diets on Energy Expenditure, Protein Metabolism and Hormone Levels in Obese Subjects." *Clinical Science* 82(1992): 85–92.

Stampfer, M.; Hennekens, C.; Manson, J.; et al. "Vitamin E Consumption and the Risk of Coronary Disease in Women." *New England Journal of Medicine* 328 (1993): 1444–49.

Ziegenfuss, T.N.; and Kerrigan, D.J. "Safety and Efficacy of Prohormone Administration in Men." Presented at 1999 Annual Meeting of American Society of Exercise Physiologists 2.

MAGIC WINDOW CONCEPT

Burke, L.M. "Nutrition for Post-Exercise Recovery." *Australian Journal of Science & Medicine in Sport* 29(1997): 3–10.

Burke, L.M.; Collier, G.R.; Davis, P.G.; et al. "Muscle Glycogen Storage After Prolonged Exercise: Effect of the Frequency of Carbohydrate Feedings." *American Journal of Clinical Nutrition* 64(1996): 115.

Doyle, J.A.; Sherman, W.M.; and Strauss, R.L. "Effects of Eccentric and Concentric Exercise on Muscle Glycogen Replenishment." *Journal of Applied Physiology.* 1993; 74(4A): 1848–55.

Pascoe, D.D.; Costill, D.L.; Fink, W.J.; et al. "Glycogen Resynthesis in Skeletal Muscle Following Resistive Exercise." *Medicine and Science in Sports and Exercise.* 1993; 25(3): 349.

Rassmussen, B.; et al. "An Oral Essential Amino Acid-Carbohydrate Supplement Enhances Muscle Protein Anabolism after Resistance Exercise." *Journal of Applied Physiology* 88(2000): 386.

Roy, B.; et al. "Macronutrient Intake and Whole Body Protein Metabolism Following Resistance Exercise." *Medicine and Science in Sports and Exercise.* 2000; 32(8): 1412.

HORMONAL EFFECTS OF EXERCISE

Braun, B.; and Horton, T. "Endocrine Regulation of Exercise Substrate and Utilization in Women Compared to Men." *Exercise and Sports Science Reviews.* 2001 Oct; 29(4): 149–54.

Cumming, D.C.; Wall, S.R.; Galbraith, M.A.; and Belcastro, A.N. "Reproductive Hormone Responses to Resistance Exercise." *Medicine and Science in Sports and Exercise.* 1987 June; 19(3): 234–38.

Elias, A.N.; and Wilson, A.F. "Exercise and Gonadal Function." *Human Reproduction.* 1993 Oct; 8(10): 1747–61.

Kraemer, W.J.; Volek, J.S.; Bush, J.A.; Putukian, M.; and Sebastianelli, W.J. "Hormonal Responses to Consecutive Days of Heavy-Resistance Exercise with or without Nutritional Supplementation." *Journal of Applied Physiology*. 1998 Oct; 85(4): 1544–55.

Marx, J.O.; Ratamess, N.A.; Nindl, B.C.; Gotshalk, L.A.; Volek, J.S.; Dohi, K.; Bush, J.A.; Gomez, A.L.; Mazzetti, S.A.; Fleck, S.J.; Hakkinen, K.; Newton, R.U.; and Kraemer, W.J. "Low-Volume Circuit Versus High-Volume Periodized Resistance Training in Women." *Medicine and Science in Sports and Exercise*. 2001 Apr; 33(4): 635–43.

Ronkainen, H.; Pakarinen, A.; Kirkinen, P.; and Kauppila, A. "Physical Exercise-Induced Changes and Season-Associated Differences in the Pituitary-Ovarian Function of Runners and Joggers." *Journal of Clinical Endocrinology and Metabolism*. 1985 Mar; 60(3): 416–22.

Tsai, L.; Karpakka, J.; Aginger, C.; Johansson, C.; Pousette, A.; and Carlstrom, K. "Basal Concentrations of Anabolic and Catabolic Hormones in Relation to Endurance Exercise after Short-Term Changes in Diet." *European Journal of Applied Physiology and Occupational Physiology*. 1993; 66(4): 304–8.

Webb, M.L.; Wallace, J.P.; Hamill, C.; Hodgson, J.L.; and Mashaly, M. "Serum Testosterone Concentration During Two Hours of Moderate Intensity Treadmill Running in Trained Men and Women." *Endocrinology Research*. 1984; 10(1): 27–38.

AEROBIC EXERCISE VERSUS WEIGHT TRAINING

Ballor, D.L.; Harvey-Berino, J.R.; Ades, P.A.; Cryan, J.; and Calles-Escandon, J. "Contrasting Effects of Resistance and Aerobic Training on Body Composition and Metabolism after Diet-Induced Weight Loss." *Metabolism*. 1996 Feb; 45(2): 179–83.

Dunn, A.L.; et al. "Six-Month Physical Activity and Fitness in Project Active: A Randomized Trial." *Medical Science Sports and Exercise*. 1998; 30(1998): 1076–83.

Geliebter, A.; Maher, M.M.; Gerace, L.; Gutin, B.; Heymsfield, S.B.; and Hashim, S.A. "Effects of Strength or Aerobic Training on Body Composition, Resting Metabolic Rate, and Peak Oxygen Consumption in Obese Dieting Subjects." *American Journal of Clinical Nutrition*. 1997 Sept; 66(3): 557–63.

Jackicic, J.M.; Winters, C.; et al. "Effect of Intermittent Exercise and Use of Home Exercise Equipment on Adherence, Weight Loss, and Fitness in Overweight Women." *Journal of the American Medical Association*. 1999 Oct 27; 282(6): 1554–60.

Wosornu, D.; Bedford, D.; and Ballantyne, D. "A Comparison of the Effects of Strength and Aerobic Exercise Training on Exercise Capacity and Lipids after Coronary Artery Bypass Surgery." *European Heart Journal.* 1996 June; 17(6): 854–63.

EATING AND MOOD/BEHAVIOR

Lieberman, H.R.; Spring, B.J.; and Garfield, G.S. "The Behavioral Effects of Food Constituents: Strategies Used in Studies of Amino Acids, Protein, Carbohydrate and Caffeine." *Nutrition Review* (44 Suppl.) (May 1986): 61–70.

Mullen, B.J.; and Martin, R.J. "The Effect of Dietary Fat on Diet Selection May Involve Central Serotonin." *American Journal of Physiology.* 1992 Sept; 263(3): Pt. 2.

Spring, B.; Chiodo, J.; and Bowen, D. "Carbohydrates, Tryptophan and Behavior: A Methodological Review." *Psychological Bulletin* 102(1987): 234–56.

Winnett, R.A. "Developing More Effective Health Behavior Programs." *Applied Preventive Psychology* 8(1998): 209–24.

Wurtman, R.J.; and Wurtman, J.J. "Brain Serotonin, Carbohydrate-Craving, Obesity and Depression." *Obesity Research.* 1995 Nov; 3(Suppl. 4): 477S–480S. Review.

MISCELLANEOUS

Davis, Devra Lee; Bradlow, H. Leon; et al. "Medical Hypothesis: Xenoestrogens as Preventable Causes of Breast Cancer." *Environmental Health Perspectives.* 1993 Oct; 101(5): 372–77.

Mori, Trevor A.; et al. "Dietary Fish as a Major Component of a Weight-Loss Diet: Effect on Serum Lipids, Glucose, and Insulin Metabolism in Overweight Hypertensive Subjects." *American Journal of Clinical Nutrition* 70(Nov. 1999): 817–25.

Pugh, T.D.; Oberley, T.D.; and Weindruch, R. "Dietary Intervention at Middle Age: Caloric Restriction But Not Dehydroepiandrosterone Sulfate Increases Lifespan and Lifetime Cancer Incidence in Mice." *Cancer Research.* 1999 Apr 1; 59(7): 1642–48.

Rosenbloom, A.L.; et al. "Emerging Epidemic of Type 2 Diabetes in Youth. Diabetes Care." 1999 Feb; 22(2): 345–54.

Ruby, B.C.; Coggan, A.R.; and Zderic, T.W. "Gender Differences in Glucose Kinetics and Substrate Oxidation During Exercise Near the Lactate Threshold." *Journal of Applied Physiology.* 2002 Mar; 92(3): 1125–32.

Skov, A.R.; et al. "Randomized Trial on Protein vs. Carbohydrates in Ad Libitum Fat-Reduced Diet for the Treatment of Obesity." *International Journal of Obesity* 23(1999): 528–36.

Spindler, S.R. "Calorie Restriction Enhances the Expression of Key Metabolic Enzymes Associated with Protein Renewal During Aging." *Annals of the New York Academy of Sciences* 928(Apr. 2001): 296–304. Review.

Weindruch, R. "The Retardation of Aging by Caloric Restriction: Studies in Rodents and Primates." *Toxicologic Pathology.* 1996 Nov-Dec; 24(6): 742–45.

INDEX

Ab crunches, 165
Abdominal muscle exercises,
    163–166
Aerobic exercise, 9, 22, 26–28
Afterburn effect, 23
Age-associated memory impairment,
    149
Aging, 106, 129
    and hormones, 134–144
    and lifestyle, 129–134
Alcohol, 131
Alzheimer's disease, 149–150
American College of Sports
    Medicine, 21
American diet, 10–11
Androdiol, 104–106
Androgel, 142
Andropausal weight gain, 139–144
Antifungal drugs, 132
Anti-inflammatory drugs, 132

Antioxidants, 98
Appetite-regulating hormone system,
    11, 13–14
Arimidex (anastrozole), 141
Aromasin (exemestane), 141
Aromatase, 8

Bakery items, 62
Benecol, 56
Benign prostate hypertrophy (BPH),
    143
Bent-leg dead lifts, 162
Bent-over rows, 160
Berries, 58
Beta-carotene, 98
Beverages, 61
Bioelectrical impedance analysis
    (BIA), 125
Black cohosh, 137
Body-fat percentage, 124–126

Body-fat scales, 123–126
Body-fat weight, 120
Brain, 28
Breakfast cereals, 54–55
Breakfast Omelet, 70–71
Breakfast recipes, 69–73
Broiled Salmon with Sesame Spinach
    and Beet Salad, 76–77
Butter, 51–52

Caffeine, 110
Calcium, 98
Calorie-tracking machines, 126–127
Cancer, 148
Carbohydrates, 6, 19
    high-fiber, 45
    low-fiber, 45–47
    Magic Window for, 42–43,
        45–47
    moderate-fiber, 45
    sources of, 46
    timing consumption of, 41–48
Cardiovascular disease, 146–147
CCK (cholecystokinin), 13, 45
Celebrex (celecoxib), 132
Cheat foods, 118
Cheese, 56
Cheesecake Cheater, 92
Chicken Curry, 82–83
Chronic fatigue, 150
Cigarettes, 131
Colds, 149
Core supplements, 97–99
Cortisol, 14, 22
Cottage cheese, 57
Creatine, 100–102
Cycling, 26

Daily eating schedule, 94–95
Dairy items, 55–57

Depression, 150–151
DEXA (dual energy X-ray
    absorptiometry), 125
DHEA (dehydroepiandrosterone),
    138–139
Diabetes, 148
Diet
    beginning, 39–41
    carbohydrate timing, 41–48
    fats, 49–52
    reality of, 6
    without starvation, 153
Diet and health foods, 62
Diflucan (fluconazole), 132
Dining out, 66–68
Dinner recipes
    poultry, 82–87
    seafood, 74–81
    side dishes, 88
Disease, fighting, 145–151
Doctor visit, 20–21
Dumbbell bench press, 161

Early-morning exercise, 23–24
Eggs, 56
Elliptical exercise machine, 26
Empty stomach, 24–25
Enbrel (etanercept), 132
Energy, 15–16
Ephedrine, 108–109
Essential fatty acids, 99
Estrogen, 7
    natural, 136–137
    toxic, 133–134, 136
Estrogen replacement therapy,
    136–137
Evolution, 5
Exercise. See Hormone Revolution
    Exercise Plan
Exercise splits, 31–32

Farmed fish, 57
Fast foods, 10–11
Fat(s), 49–52
    healthy, 49–51
    omega-6 fatty acids, 51
    sources of, 50
    storage of, 5
    unhealthy, 51–52
Fat cells, 29
Fat-Free Chicken Sandwich, 89
FDA (Food and Drug Administration), 108–109
Femara (letrozole), 141
Fiber, 44
Fiber One, 55
Fish oil, 99
Flaxseed oil, 99
Flu, 149
Forskolin, 111
Four-day exercise plan, 35
Free weights, 29
Fruit, 47, 58, 59
Fruit juice, 47
Fruit Salad with Shrimp, 71–72

Garlic-Pepper Chicken Breasts, 85
Glucose, 10
Grains, 88
Gravity, 26–27, 29
Green tea, 110–111
Grilled Halibut Salad, 77–78
Grocery selections, 54
    bakery section, 62
    beverage section, 61
    breakfast cereal aisle, 54–55
    dairy aisle, 55–57
    diet and health food aisle, 62
    meat and seafood counter, 57, 58
    produce section, 58, 59
    snacks and sweets aisle, 63

Guarana, 110
Guilt-Free Teriyaki Chicken, 87
Gym, 21

HDL cholesterol, 104, 146
Health Canada, 109–110
Healthy fats, 49–51
Heart disease, 146–147
Herbs, 59–61
High-Powered Protein Shake, 90
High-Protein Blueberry Pancakes, 72–73
High pulls, 162
Hormone(s)
    and aging, 134–144
    appetite-regulating, 13–14
    growth, 11–12
    harnessing, 6–7
    insulin system, 10–11
    and lifestyle, 14–16
    metabolic, 12–13
    sex, 7–10
Hormone boosters, 99–106
Hormone replacement therapy, 135
Hormone Revolution Eating Plan, 39–95
    beginning diet, 39–41
    carbohydrate timing and Magic Window, 41–48
    daily eating schedules, 94–95
    fats and protein, 48–54
    food log for, 118–119
    grocery selections, 54–63
    implementing, 63–68
    recipes, 68–92
    troubleshooting, 121–123
    vegetarian cooking, 92–93
    weighing in, 119–120

Hormone Revolution Exercise Plan, 19–38
abdominal muscle exercises, 163–166
aerobic exercise, 26–28
beginning, 19–22
exercise log for, 115–116
exercise splits, 31–32
lower-body exercises, 162–163
"non-exercise" exercise, 37–38
periodization, 32–34
sample schedules, 34–37
timing, 23–25
troubleshooting, 116–117
upper-body exercises, 159–161
weight-lifting instructions, 158–163
weight training, 28–30
Hormone Revolution Supplement Plan, 96–113
core supplements, 97–99
hormone boosters, 99–106
thermogenics, 106–113
Hormone Revolution Weight-Loss Plan, 16–18
Human growth hormone, 11–12, 133, 143

Immune system, 149
Injuries, 117–118
Insomnia, 122
Insulin, 23–24, 148
Insulin system, 10–11
Internet, 127–128
Isoflavones, 137

Junk foods, 10–11

Lamisil (terbinafine hydrochloride), 132

Large muscle groups, 31
Lateral raises, 160–161
Lateral twists, 165–166
LDL cholesterol, 146
Lean body weight, 120
Leptin, 29
Libido, 16
Life extension, 154–155
Life span, 8
Lifestyle and aging, 14–16, 129
medication, 131–132
sleep, 132–133
stress, 130–131
Lifetime Specialty Cheeses, 56
Lime Salmon, 80
Low-Carb Breaded Fried Chicken, 86
Low-carbohydrate diet, 10, 41
Lower-body exercises, 162–163
Lunch recipes
poultry, 82–87
seafood, 74–81
side dishes, 88
Lunge Squats, 163

Ma huang, 109–110
Magic Window, 13, 42–43, 45–47, 62–63, 65–66
side dishes, 88–89
Magnesium, 98
Male androgen insufficiency syndrome, 139
Margarine, 51–52, 56
Max lift, 30
McCann's Irish Oatmeal, 55
Meat, 57, 58
Meat and seafood, 57, 58
Medications, 15, 131–132
Mediterranean diet, 68
Memory impairment, 149–150

Men
    rising estrogen levels in, 8
Menopausal weight gain, 135–139
Metabolism, 12–13, 23
Monitoring success, 114
    dietary progress
        food log, 118–119
    exercise progress
        exercise log, 115–116
        injuries and role of physical
            therapy, 117–118
        troubleshooting, 116–117
    technology
        body-fat scales, 123–126
        calorie-tracking machines,
            126–127
        Internet, 127–128
        troubleshooting, 121–123
    weighing in, 119–120
    weight-loss plateaus, 114–115
Monounsaturated fats, 49
Multivitamin/multimineral
    formulas, 97–99
Muscle
    preservation, 5–6
    prolonged soreness in, 116–117
    protein as building block of, 53

Nicotine, 131
Nizoral (ketoconazole), 132
Nonfat milk products, 66
Nutty Cottage Cheese, 91

Okinawan women, 67
Olive oil, 49
Omega-3 fatty acids, 49–50, 57, 99
Omega-6 fatty acids, 51
Osteoporosis, 29, 147

Partially hydrogenated oils, 52
Periodization of exercise, 32–34

Personal trainer, 21
Personalized program, 156–157
Phen-fen, 14
Phosphatidyl serine, 102–103
Physical therapy, 117–118
Phytoestrogens, 136–137
Phytonutrients, 148
Pilates exercise system, 26–27
Plateau lift, 30
Polyphenols, 111
Postmenopausal women, testosterone
    decrease in, 8–9
Prednisone, 132
Premarin, 136
Prevacid (lansoprazole), 132
Processed foods, 10–11
Produce, 58, 59
Progesterone, 136
Prohormones, 104
Promise, 56
Protein, 6, 52–54
    sources of, 53
Protein shake, 53–54
Provera, 136–137
Pyramid, 33

Recipes
    breakfast, 69–73
    lunch and dinner
        poultry, 82–87
        seafood, 74–81
        side dishes, 88
        snacks, 89–92
Recommended Daily Allowance
    (RDA), 98
Relaxation, 152
Reproductive age, 8
Resources, 167–173
Rest-growth period, 31
Reverse crunches, 164
Reverse pyramid, 33

Salads, 88
Salt, 60
Sauces, 59–61
Seafood, 57, 58, 74–81
Seared Ahi Tuna, 75
Sex, 151–153
Sex hormones, 7–10
Side dishes, 88–89
Six-day exercise plan, 36
Sleep, 15, 132–133, 152–153
Smoking, 131
Snacks, 66, 89–92
Snacks and sweets, 63
Soy, 137
Soy sauce, 61
Soymilk, 55–56
Spices, 59–61
Stair climbers, 27
Standard meal, 64, 65
Standing biceps dumbbell curls, 159
Standing exercise, 29–30
Starches, 10–11, 47, 150
Starvation, 9, 48, 122, 153
Stress, 14–15, 130–131
Sugar, 150
Sweets, 47
Swimming, 26
Synephrine, 109

Tagamet (cimetidine), 132
Testosterone, 8, 22–23, 104, 132,
    137–139
  safety of, 143–144
Testosterone replacement therapy,
    141–142
Thermic effect, 52
Thermogenics, 106–113
  benefits of, 107–108
  forskolin, 111
  green tea, 110–111
  guarana, 110

how to use, 111–113
  ma huang, 109–110
  precautions for, 108–109
Three-day split exercises, 32
Thyroid hormone, 12–13
Timing exercise, 23–25
Total body-fat weight, 120
Training buddy, 22
Trans-fatty acids, 11, 51
Treadmill, inclined, 26–27
Tri-Orange Roughy, 79
Two-day split exercises, 31–32

Ulcer medications, 132
Unhealthy fats, 51–52
Upper-body exercises, 159–161

Vegetables, 58, 59, 88
Vegetarian cooking, 92–93
Vitamin A, 98
Vitamin C, 98
Vitamin E, 98

Warm-up set, 30
Watercress, Pear, and Walnut Salad
    with Poppy Seed Dressing,
    83–84
Weight-lifting instructions, 158–163
Weight-lifting machines, 33
Weight-loss plateaus, 114–115
Weight training, 28–30
  plus aerobic periodization, 34
Whey protein, 53
White foods, 45, 62

Xenoestrogens, 133–134

Yogurt, 56–57

Zesty Tomato Fish, 81
Zinc, 98